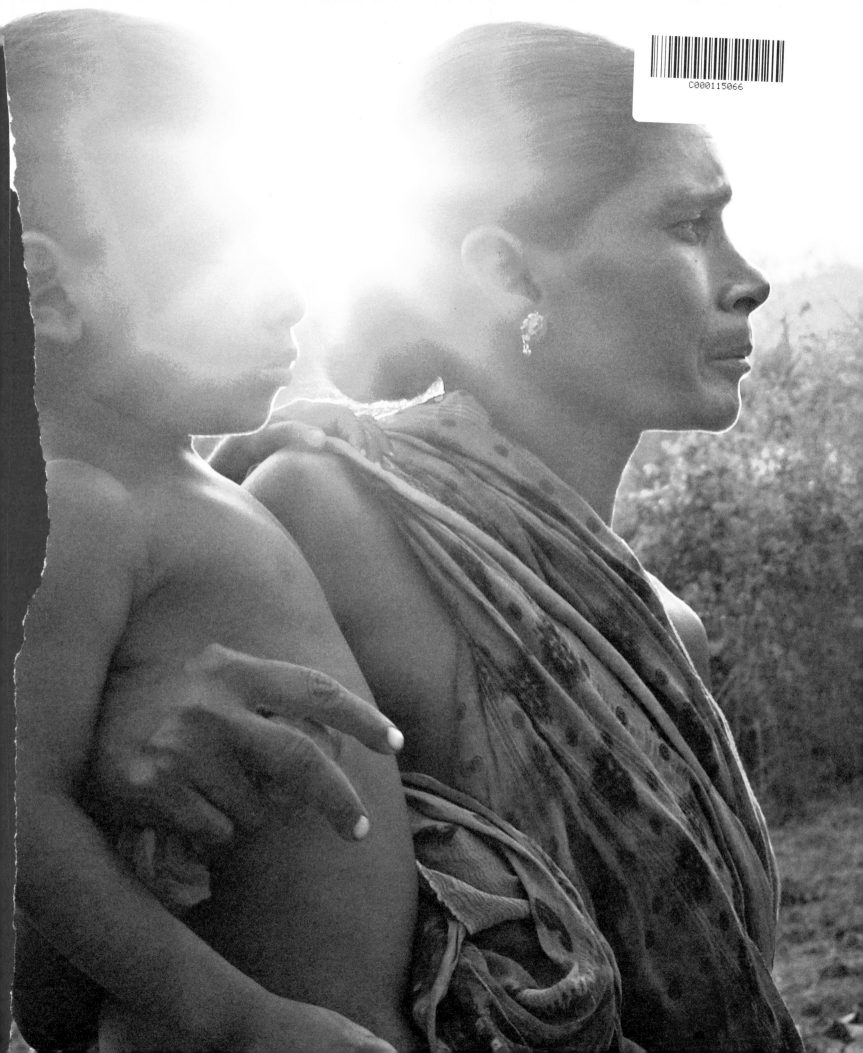

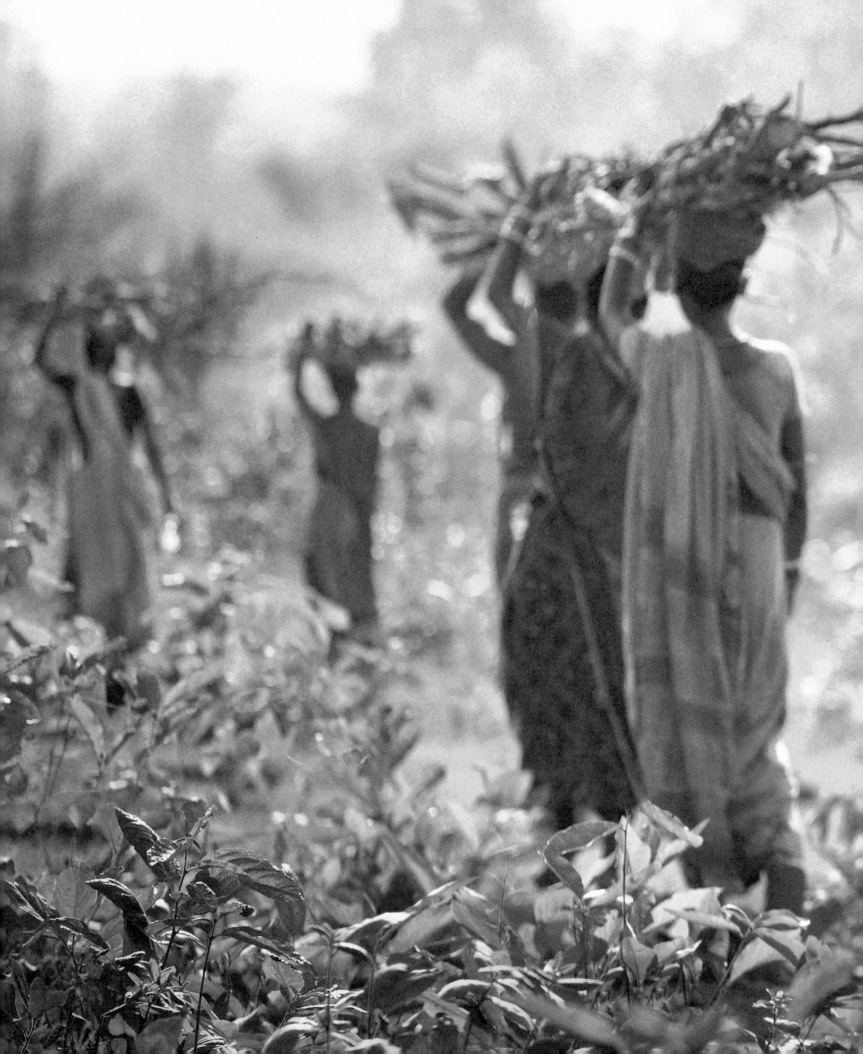

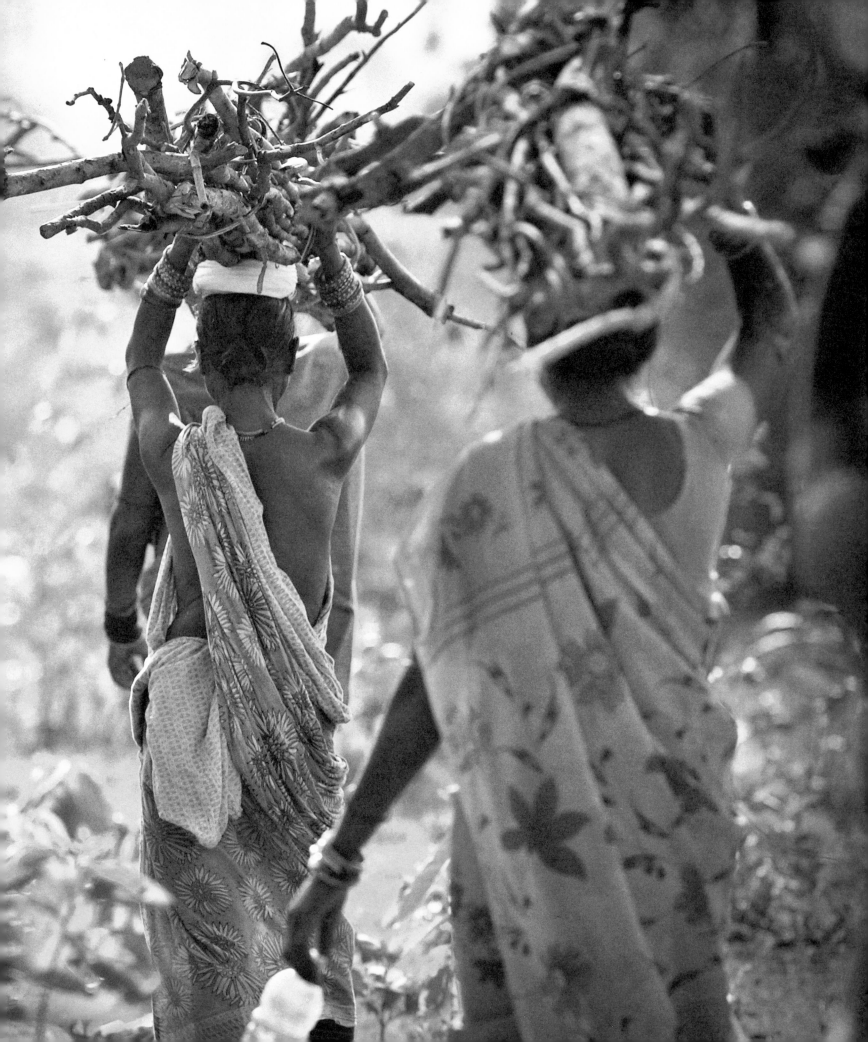

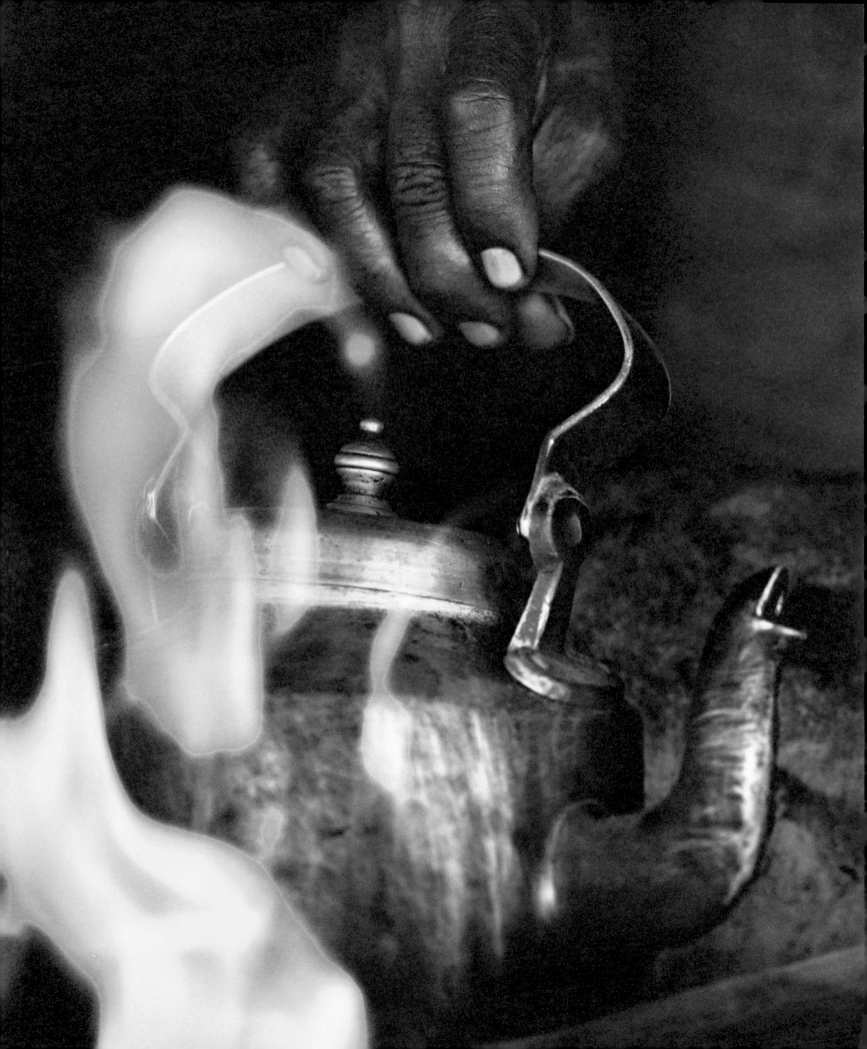

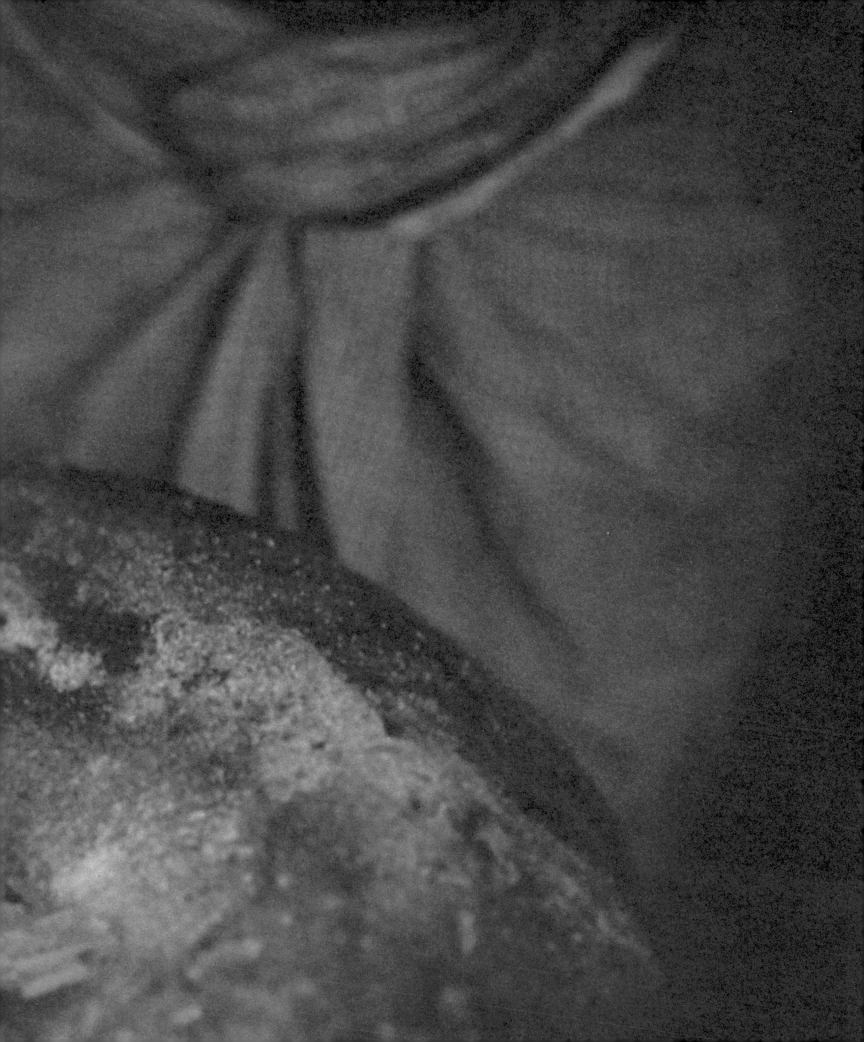

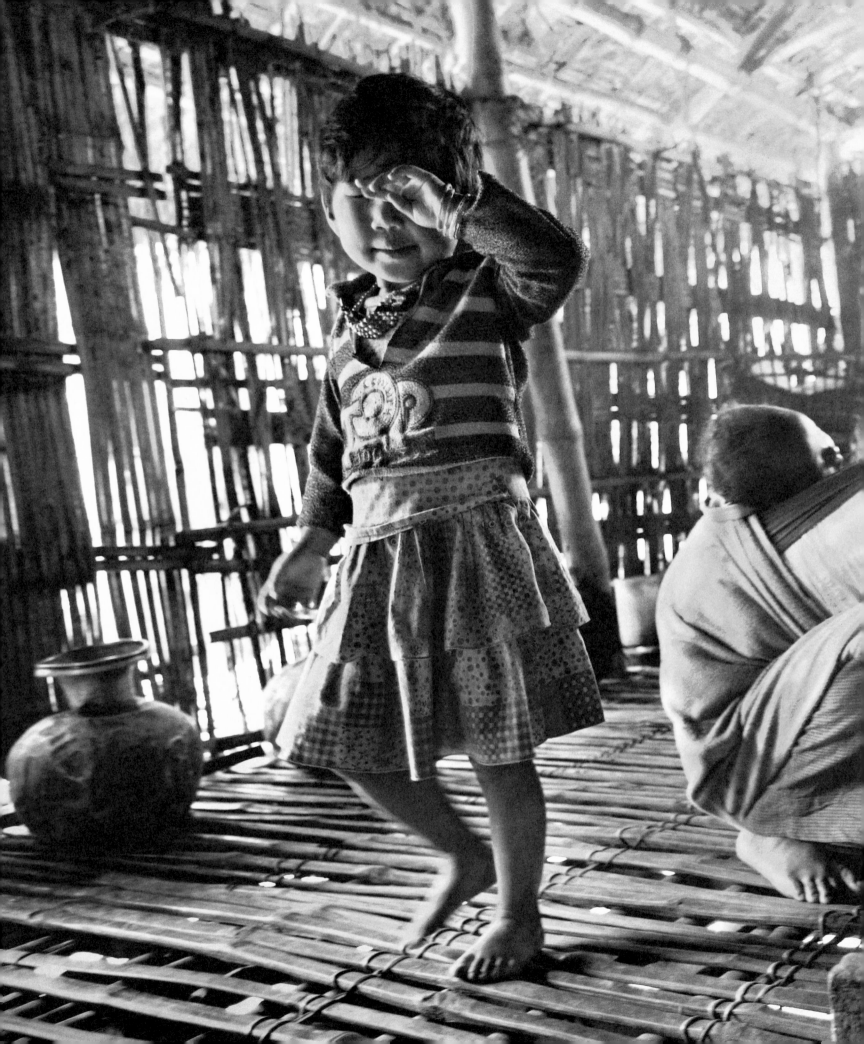

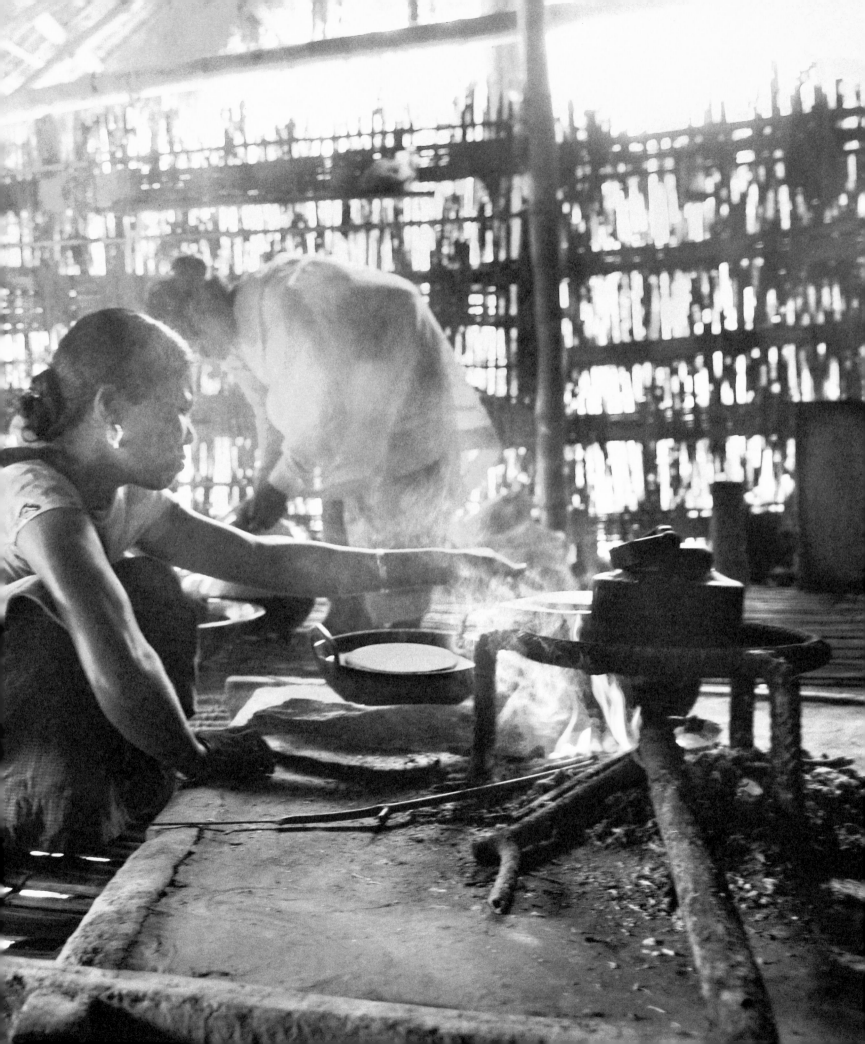

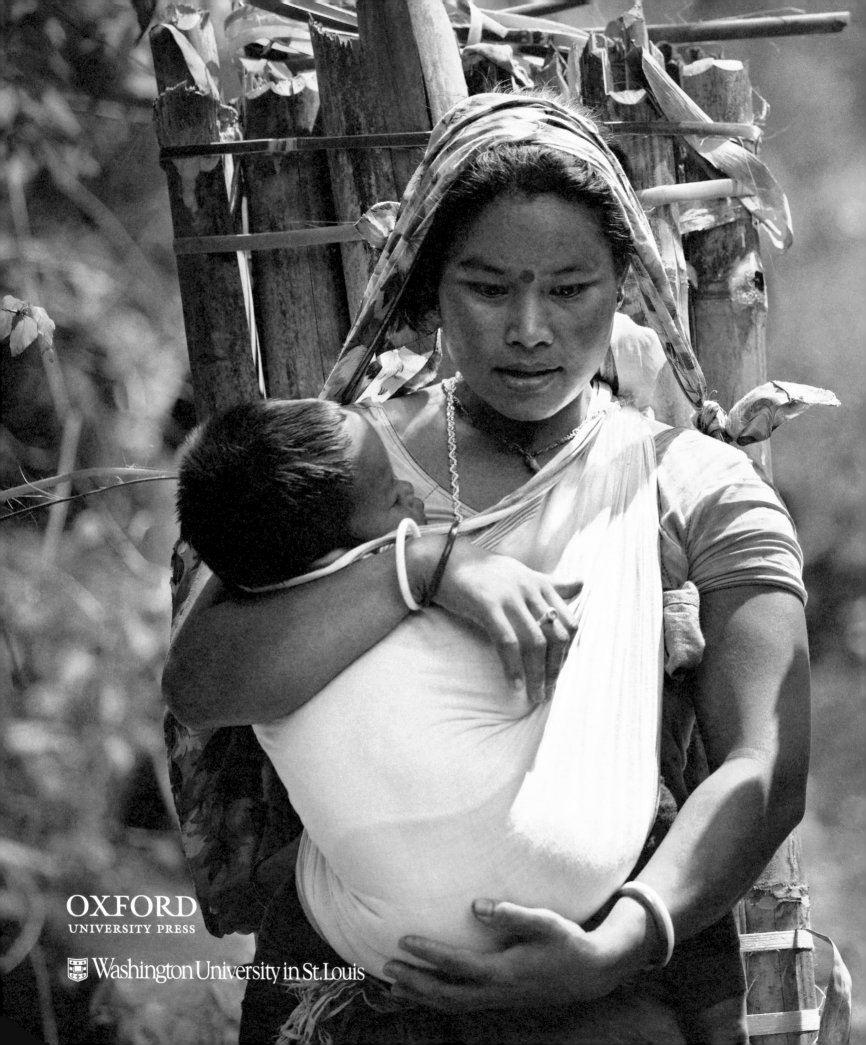

FIRES, FUEL & THE FATE OF 3 BILLION

THE STATE OF THE ENERGY IMPOVERISHED

GAUTAM N. YADAMA

PHOTOGRAPHS BY MARK KATZMAN

WITH CONTRIBUTIONS FROM

Pratim Biswas, Brent Williams, Tiffany Knight, Nishesh Chalise, Mario Castro, and the Foundation for Ecological Security, India

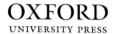

OXFORD
UNIVERSITY PRESS

Oxford University Press is a department of the University of Oxford. It furthers the University's objective of excellence in research, scholarship, and education by publishing worldwide.

Oxford New York
Auckland Cape Town Dar es Salaam Hong Kong Karachi
Kuala Lumpur Madrid Melbourne Mexico City Nairobi
New Delhi Shanghai Taipei Toronto

WITH OFFICES IN
Argentina Austria Brazil Chile Czech Republic France Greece
Guatemala Hungary Italy Japan Poland Portugal Singapore
South Korea Switzerland Thailand Turkey Ukraine Vietnam

Oxford is a registered trademark of Oxford University Press in the UK and certain other countries.

PUBLISHED IN THE UNITED STATES OF AMERICA BY
Oxford University Press
198 Madison Avenue, New York, NY 10016

EDITORIAL DIRECTION AND DESIGN BY
TOKY (toky.com); typeset in the Odile, National, and Knockout type families; printed on Mohawk Options 100PC White Smooth; produced in an edition of 1,250.

LIBRARY OF CONGRESS CATALOGING-IN-PUBLICATION DATA
Yadama, Gautam N.
Fires, Fuel, and the Fate of 3 Billion: The State of the Energy Impoverished / Gautam N. Yadama; photographs by Mark Katzman.
Pages cm
Includes bibliographical references.
ISBN 978-0-19-933667-8
1. Poor families—India. 2. Fuel—India. 3. Household appliances—Energy conservation—India.
4. Sex role—India. 5. Women—India—Social conditions. I. Title.
HC440.P5Y33 2013
333.79'630954—dc23
2013017004

9 8 7 6 5 4 3 2 1

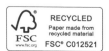

Washington University in St. Louis   TOKY BRANDING + DESIGN

Printed in China on acid-free paper

For Y.S. Rao (Yadama Sudhakara Rao)

AUTHOR'S NOTE

This book has two primary parts: first, a central essay outlining the issue of energy
impoverishment, using India as a case study to convey the predicament of 3 billion people
on this planet; and second, a series of five narratives that documents how this complex
issue is at play in the lives of individual communities in different parts of India. Decisions,
alternatives, and livelihoods in these narratives illustrate why energy choices are an
outcome of interacting forces from within and outside the command of the energy poor.

As this book is a call for a more transdisciplinary approach, throughout you will see
occasional sidebars providing insights by experts in their fields (ecology and engineering,
for example). The endnotes for all sources are listed after the Epilogue, numbered and
categorized by book section.

Mark Katzman's photographs, which vividly illustrate each part of this book, were
taken during 2011 and 2012 in many of the same communities in which my research,
in collaboration with the Foundation for Ecological Security, has been unfolding during
the past half-decade.

Thank you. —G.Y.

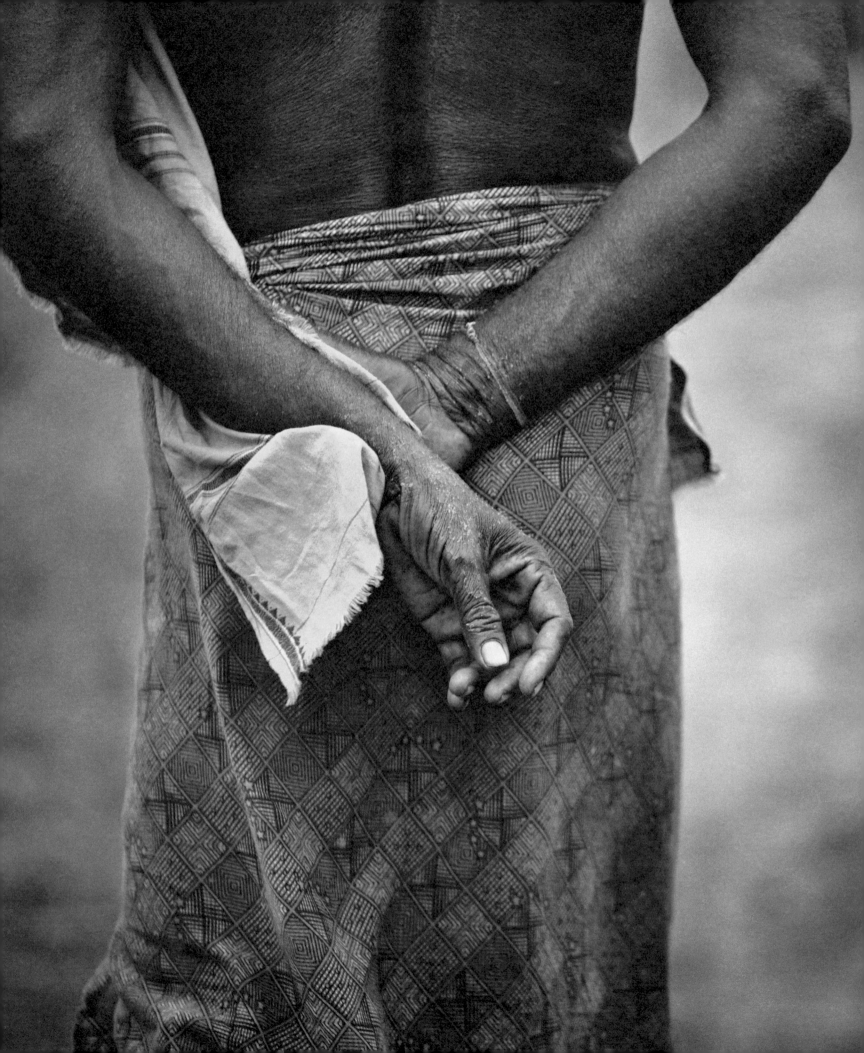

CONTENTS

15   Foreword by Director General Kandeh Yumkella

16   Foreword by Chancellor Mark S. Wrighton

19   Prologue

36   The Energy Impoverished:
       *Seeking a Greater Understanding
       of a Complex and Wicked Problem*

66   Narrative One: Women, Wood & Burning
       Patchwork Lives in the Satkosia Gorge

80   Narrative Two: Land & Living
       The Paradox of Kutch

96   Narrative Three: Stalled by Tradition
       Energy on the Islands of Brahmaputra

110   Narrative Four: Cause & Effect
       Feedback Loops in Andhra Pradesh and Rajasthan

128   Narrative Five: Searching for Agency
       The Power of People and Communities

147   Epilogue

151   Endnotes

156   Acknowledgments

FOREWORD

Energy is essential for development.

As UN Secretary-General Ban Ki-moon has often said, "Energy is the golden thread that connects economic growth, increased social equity, and an environment that allows the world to thrive." Access to modern energy services is a prerequisite to the achievement of all of the Millennium Development Goals—from supporting a child's education and reducing maternal and child mortality to improving agriculture, fostering gender equality, and enhancing environmental sustainability.

This book illustrates how access to modern energy services can transform people's lives in households and communities around the world. The stories told here are not unique to the Indian context. They are representative of the struggles faced by so many families across the globe. Currently, nearly 3 billion people lack access to clean-cooking solutions, and the smoke from their fires and kerosene-based lighting contributes to indoor air pollution that kills millions of women and children annually. Their lack of modern energy services has a profoundly negative impact on their environment, their economy, and even their safety. *Fires, Fuel, and the Fate of 3 Billion* personalizes this problem and gives it a human face, indeed a woman's face, and amplifies the voices of those for whom energy remains a critical need in the second decade of the 21st century.

The UN Secretary-General's initiative on Sustainable Energy for All (SE4ALL) has adopted universal access to modern energy services in all of its dimensions—clean cooking, electrification, and heating—as one of three global objectives to be reached by 2030. Leading worldwide efforts to enhance access to and adoption of clean-cooking solutions is the Global Alliance for Clean Cookstoves, a public-private partnership of hundreds of organizations led by the UN Foundation. With the outcome document of the Rio+20 Summit stressing the importance of energy services to sustainable development, and the unanimous declaration by UN Member States of a Decade of Sustainable Energy for All, beginning in 2014, energy issues—and their solutions—will rightly be at the forefront of the international sustainable development agenda for years to come.

The importance of building local markets for solutions must be underscored in this effort. Strong markets are critical to ensuring deployment of high-quality, well-maintained solutions that provide a lasting benefit to poor people in their daily lives.

With stunning visuals, cogent analysis, and moving testimonials, this important book calls us to hear the collective voice of those most affected by energy poverty, to "build respectful trading zones of knowledge" among users and designers, and to provide sustainable and affordable solutions, so that in the future—in all countries affected by energy poverty—no woman has to walk eight hours or sacrifice her health to cook the food needed to feed her family.

KANDEH K. YUMKELLA, PH.D.
Director General, United Nations Industrial Development Organization (UNIDO)
Special Representative of the Secretary General & Chief Executive,
Sustainable Energy for All (SE4All)

FOREWORD

Securing abundant, affordable energy while minimizing adverse effects on the environment is a global imperative. Leaders in the scientific and educational communities have stressed this point over and over during the past several decades, with a focus primarily on the massive global thirst for electricity and fossil fuels.

Yet for hundreds of millions of people around the world, energy resources remain scarce. Energy access has become the dividing line between the haves and the have-nots, and on one side of the line are those destined to lives of devastating poverty.

In *Fires, Fuel, and the Fate of 3 Billion: The State of the Energy Impoverished*, Washington University Professor Gautam Yadama and photographer Mark Katzman tell an eye-opening, insightful story about energy access in the rural villages of India, where the hunt for safe, affordable energy rages on as a matter of life and death. It's a story about cookstoves and fuel, but it's about so much more than that. It's about energy impoverishment, a "complex and wicked problem" with staggering consequences. The photographs and details in this book provide a palpable sense of the social norms and their burdens on women. The book offers a fresh perspective on social systems, poverty, gender roles, traditions, and ecology.

In rural India, countless numbers of women and children walk for hours each day to secure fuelwood or resort to burning crop residue, charcoal, and animal dung to feed small cookstoves and keep their homes and their families alive. "If there is no fire in the house, it is not a house," says one woman on Majuli Island, Assam. This struggle is about dignity and self-reliance. This struggle for energy is not just in India, but also in other regions of Asia and Sub-Saharan Africa.

The complex story of cookstoves in India and elsewhere is one that many have tried to understand, but it is not just about inventing a better, more efficient, and safer stove. If it were, the problem would have been solved long ago.

"Complex and wicked" problems require nuanced and interwoven solutions, and this is exactly the role and power of research universities around the world. Dr. Yadama is a professor of social work, but improving lives in India and in other developing countries will require innovative ideas from many others, including engineers, healthcare professionals, and scientists from a wide variety of fields, all working closely with communities to bring about change.

Fires, Fuel, and the Fate of 3 Billion is an introduction to a problem and a call for solutions to clear the hurdles to the adoption of new technologies that will help transition millions of people away from their reliance on traditional fuel sources and dangerous, antiquated technology.

The path to success in this endeavor lies in the hands of many people, including the innovative thinkers of today's research universities, who have a passion for taking on large global challenges and the willingness and ability to collaborate across disciplines and cultures to find solutions. This book brings home the reality of a global crisis, and it encourages solutions that lie within our reach, if we can only work together.

MARK S. WRIGHTON, PH.D.
Chancellor and Professor of Chemistry
Washington University in St. Louis

Every day, inside small homes and huts throughout the developing world, billions of people strike matches, light fires, prepare meals, heat their homes. The rudimentary stoves they use burn biomass like firewood, crop residue, charcoal, and animal dung, releasing dense black soot into their homes and the environment.

THIS STOVE TELLS A STORY

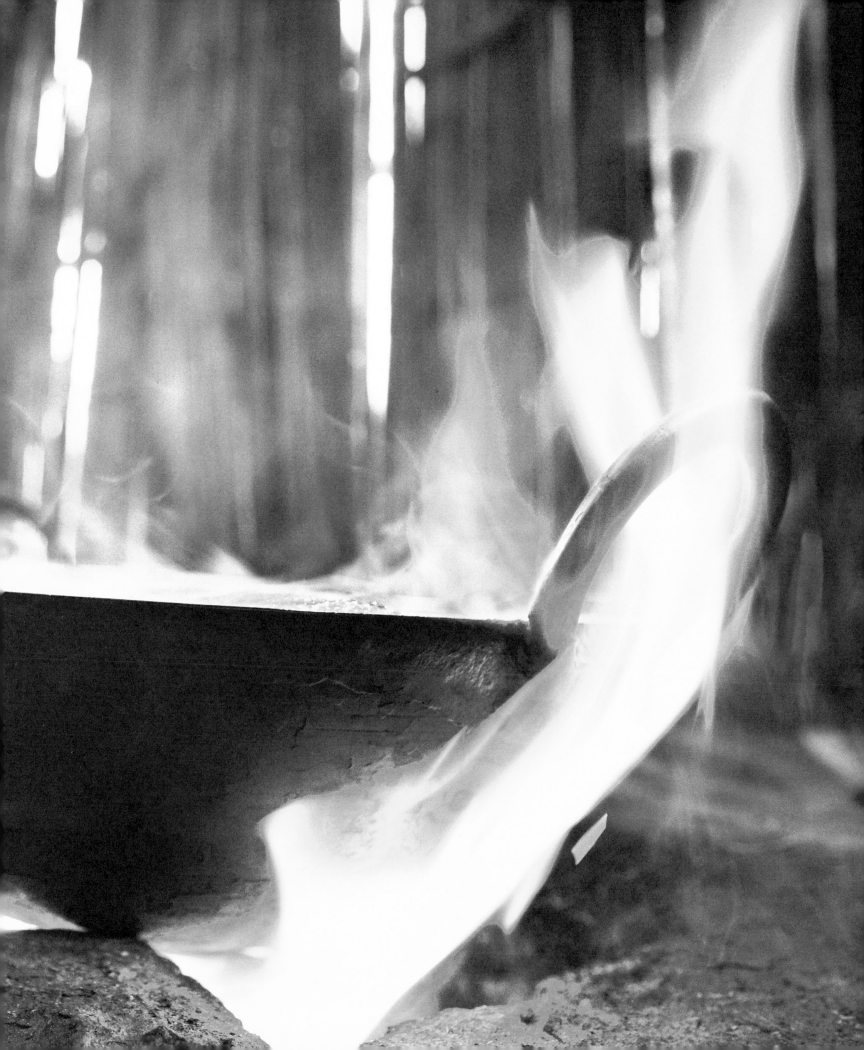

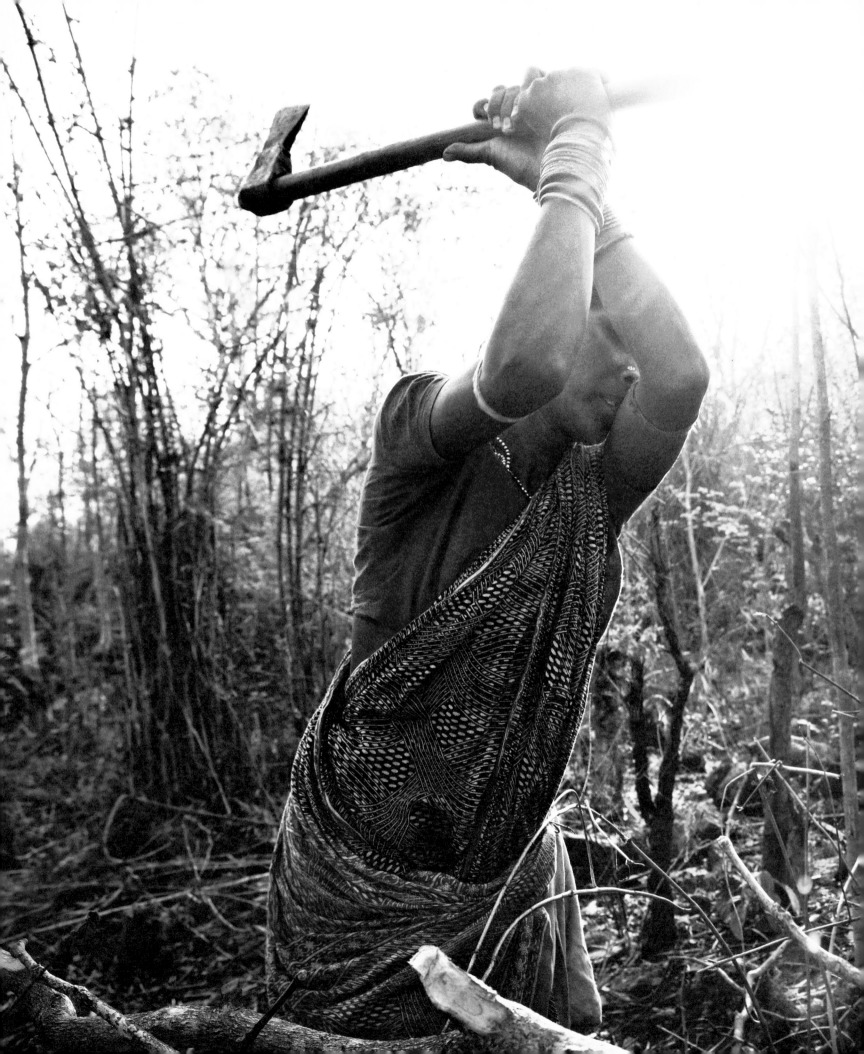

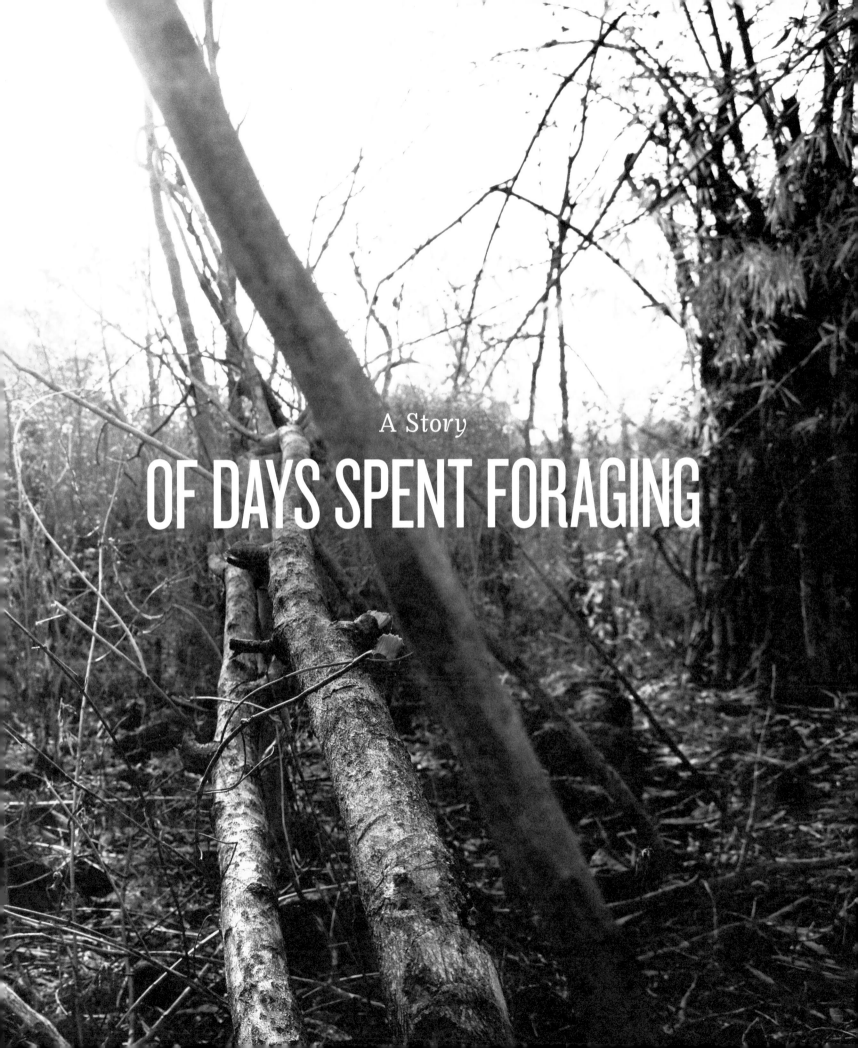

A Story

OF DAYS SPENT FORAGING

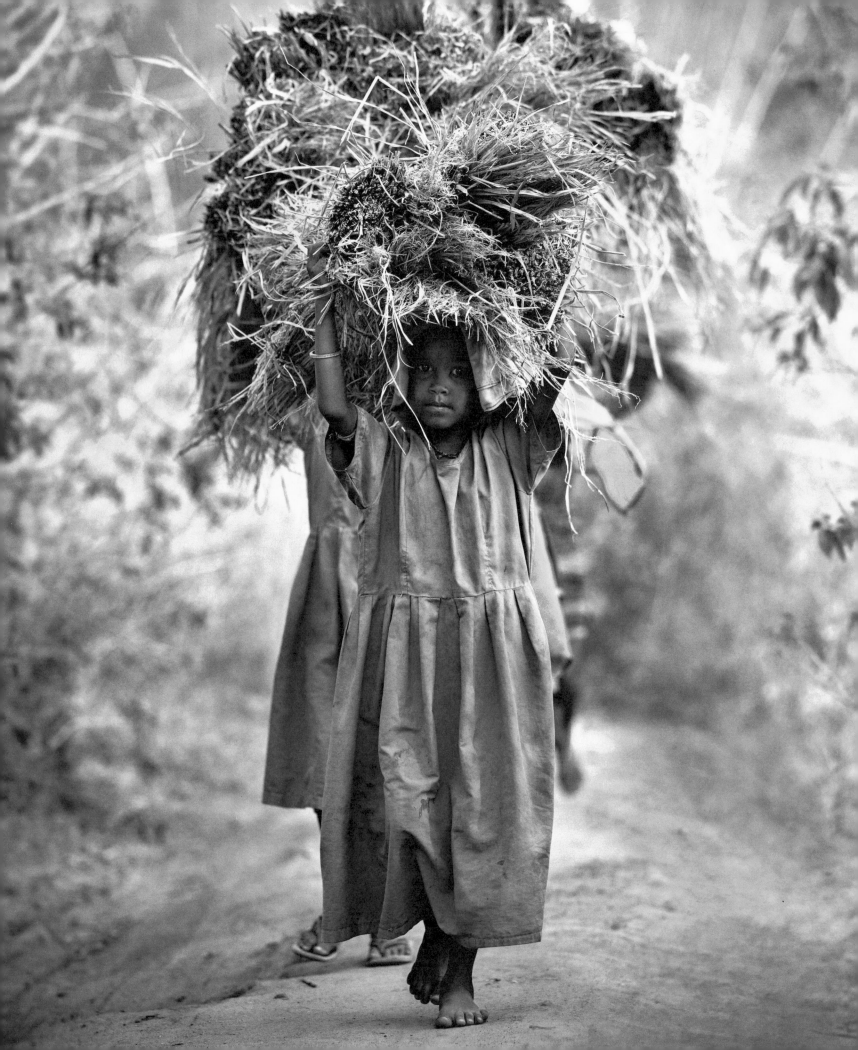

A Story

OF CHILDREN AT WORK

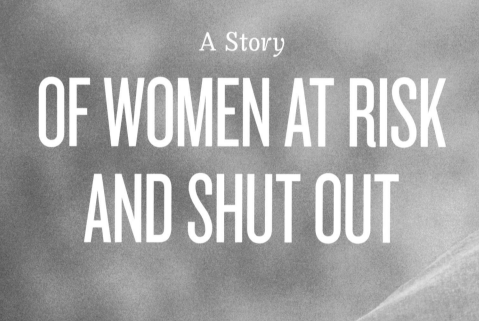

A Story

OF WOMEN AT RISK
AND SHUT OUT

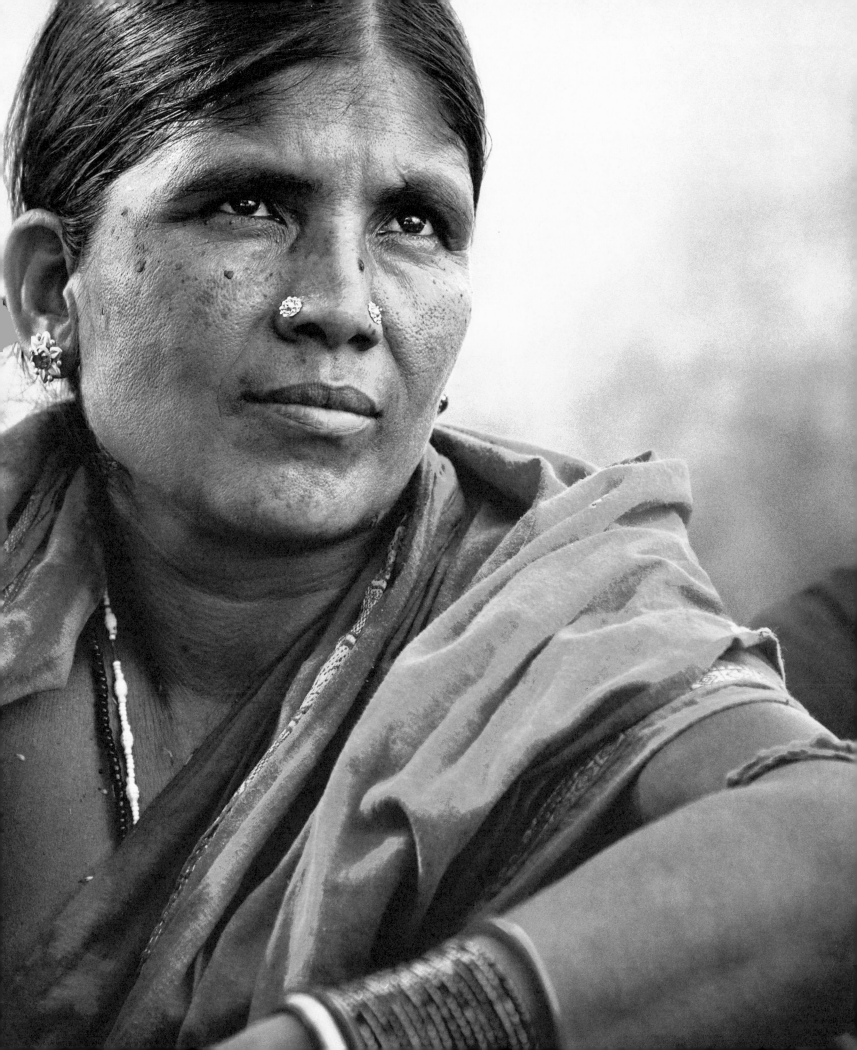

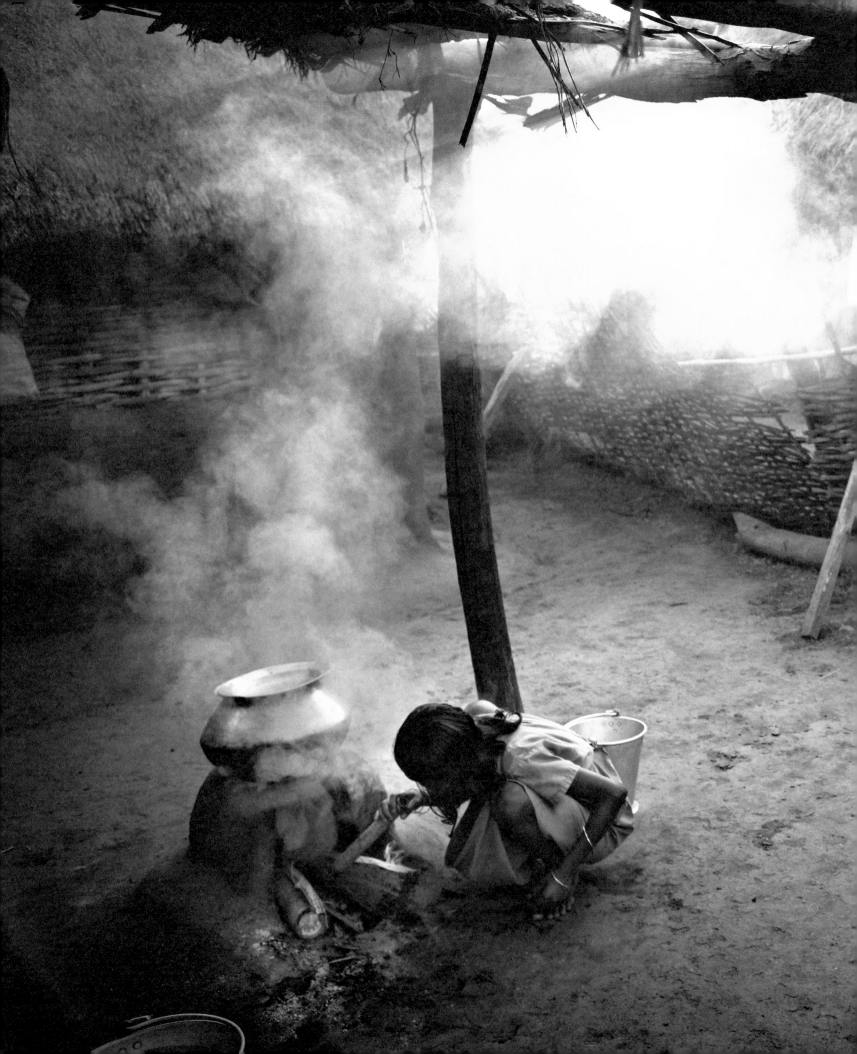

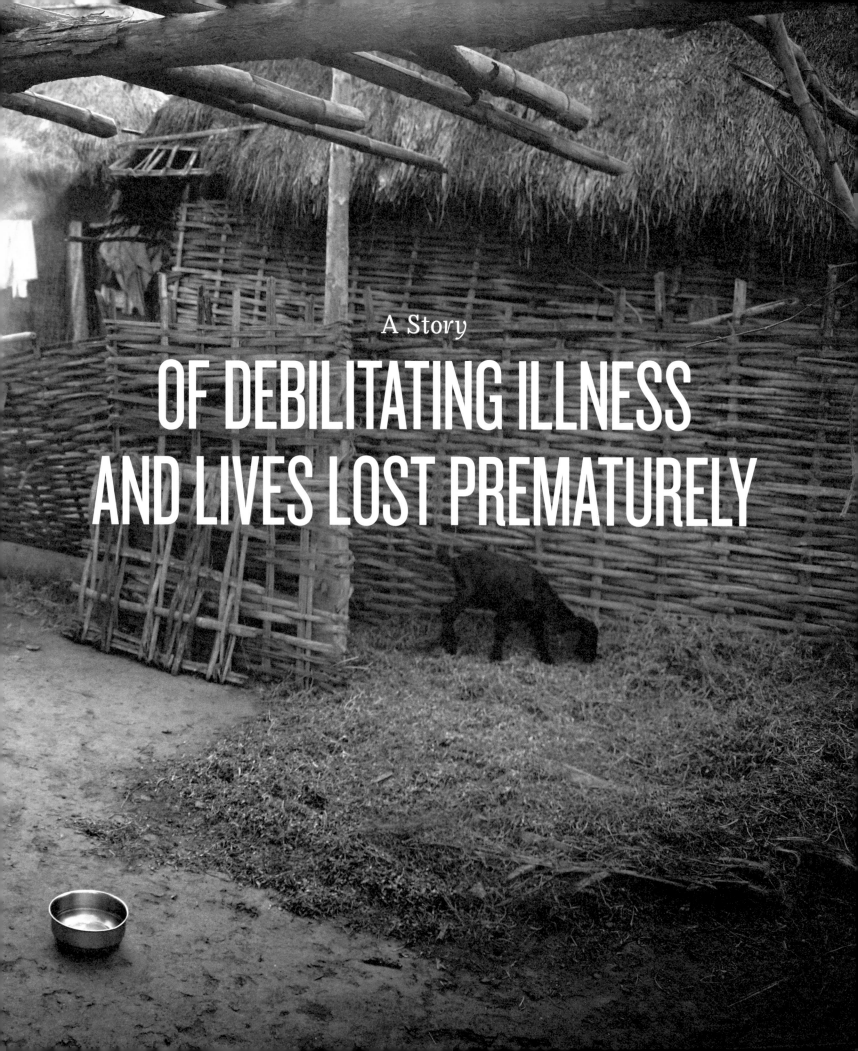

A Story

OF DEBILITATING ILLNESS AND LIVES LOST PREMATURELY

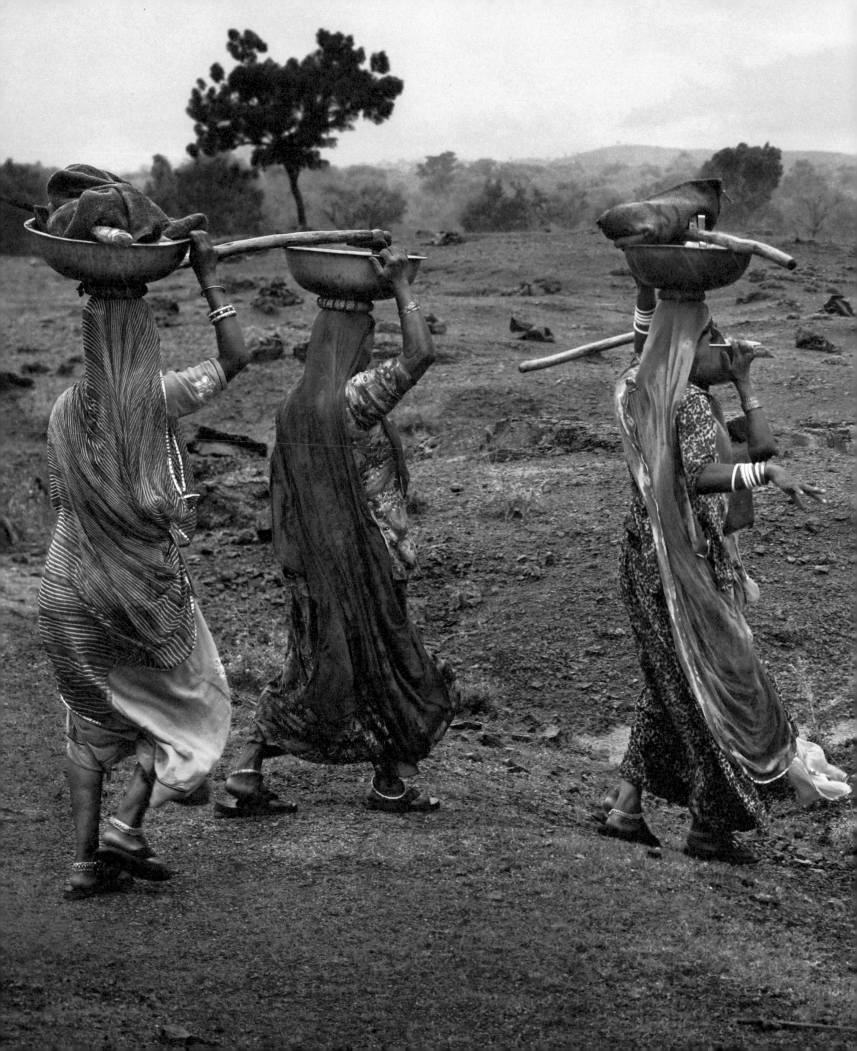

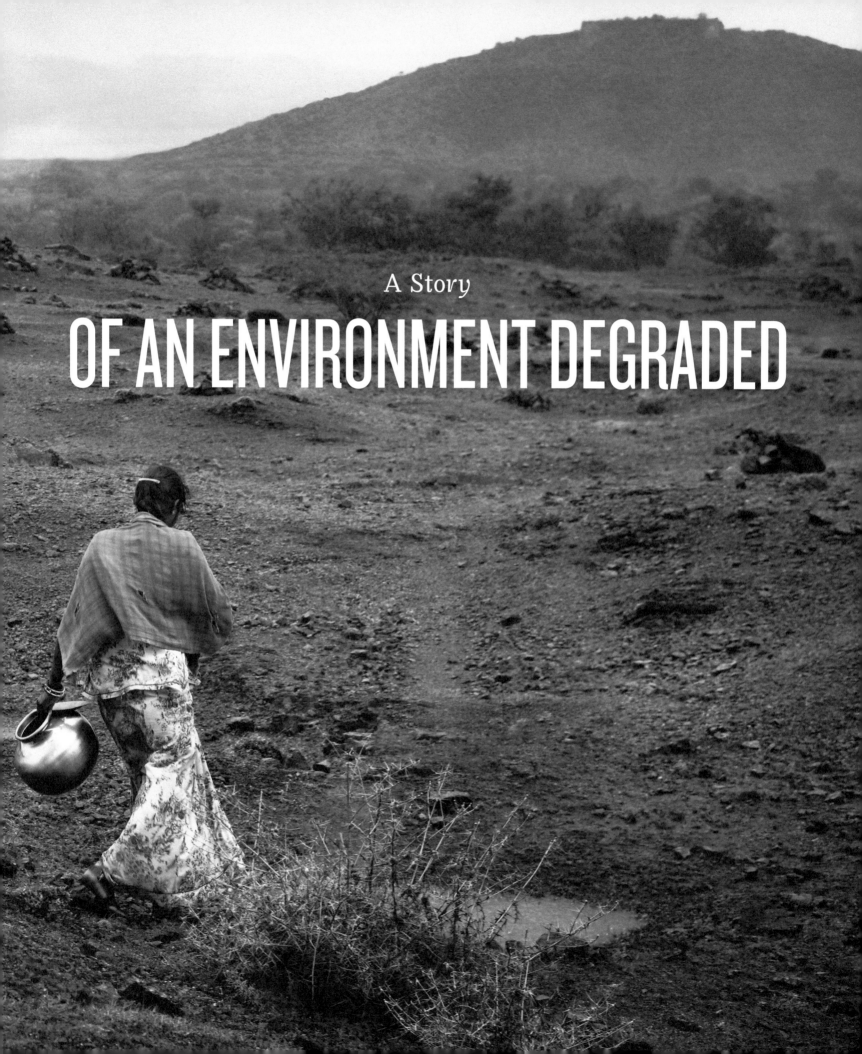

A Story

OF AN ENVIRONMENT DEGRADED

A Story

OF MULTIPLE DILEMMAS
CONVERGING AT ONCE

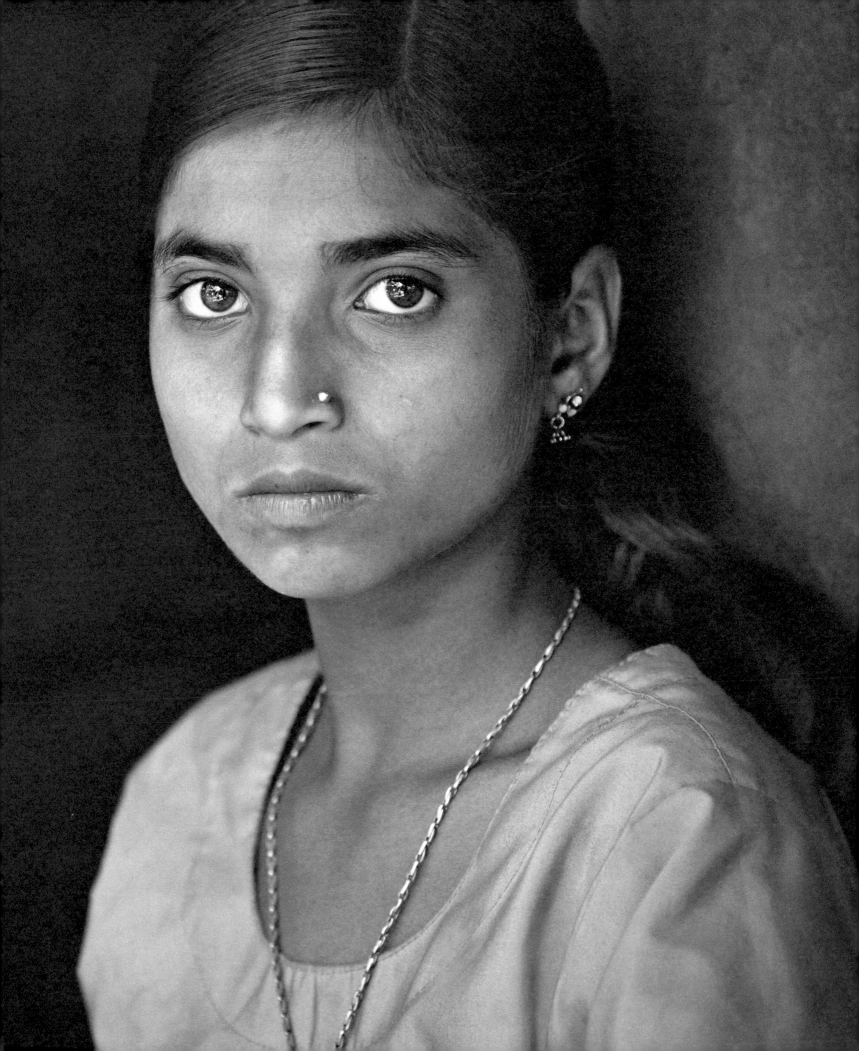

Every part of this process—from the hunt
for fuel to its daily burning—has staggering
consequences.

To understand such a vexing problem,
what must we know? Where must we go?
To whom must we listen?

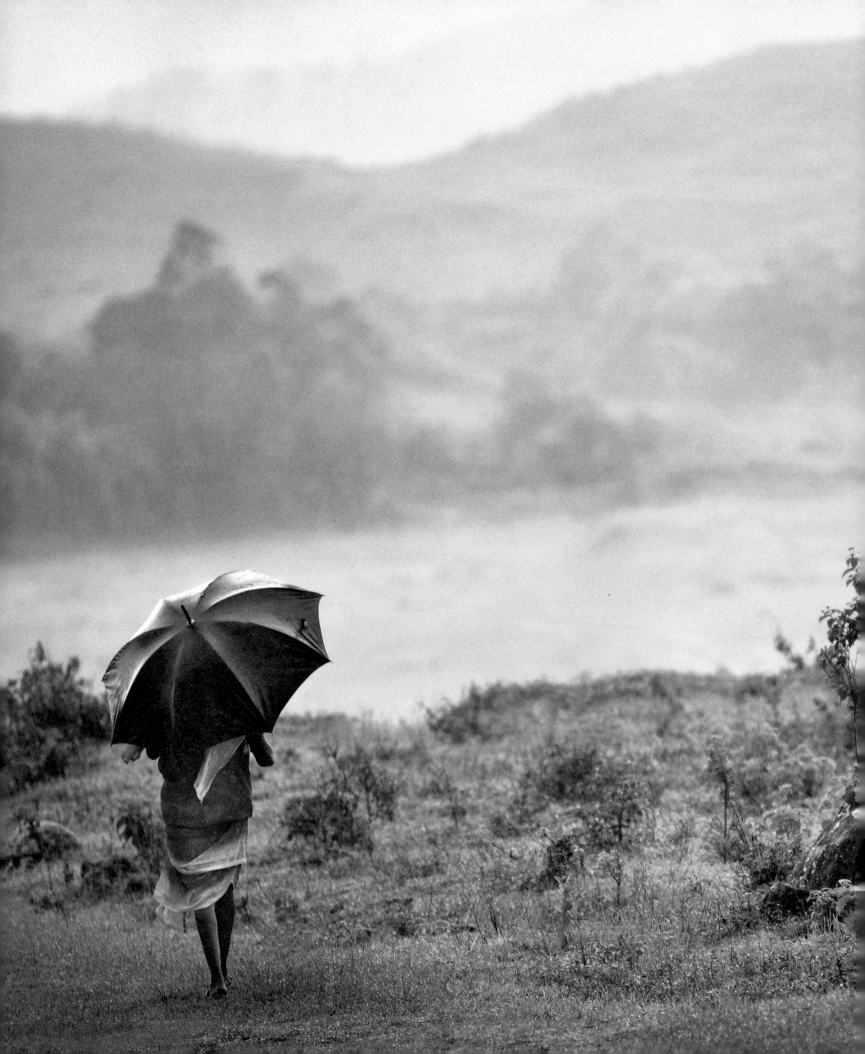

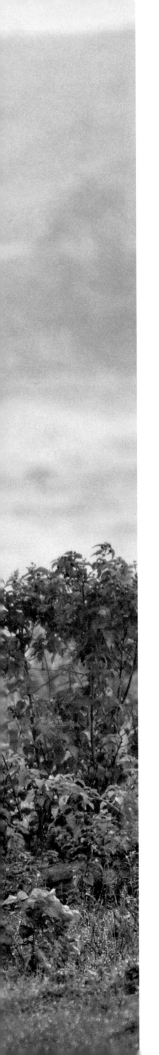

The Energy Impoverished:
Seeking a Greater Understanding
of a Complex and Wicked Problem

ONE WOMAN AMID MANY

It was July 2011, and all of Orissa was in a monsoon way. Koraput district was no exception; paddy fields and forested hills in the distance were bursting in shades of green brought by the summer rain.

Within that green was a young woman in her early 20s, dressed in a blue nightgown with white polka dots. She walked out of the forest, down a hill, head-loading thirty kilos of wood, all the while smiling and joking. It was midday.

There were twelve other women with her, also head-loading, some carrying up to fifty kilos, walking hurriedly toward home. Suddenly, they stopped, unloading the wood by the side of the road. First came the lighter bundles, fifteen or twenty kilos in weight, thrown down from their heads. Women with heavier loads carefully lowered them with help from others in the group. This was a brief rest en route to their village, seven kilometers away.

Except for the woman in polka dots, they were all from the same tribal village in the Koraput district of Orissa. She was from the neighboring state of Andhra Pradesh; here visiting her sister, she helped the entire group collect fuelwood.

She spoke Telugu, my mother tongue, and we talked about where the women were from, how far they had gone to collect wood, and how far they were from their village.

I asked this woman why she was carrying wood on her time away from home.

She answered: "A woman's fate is to carry these burdens. Is it not our sole purpose of living? Our life is meant for this alone."

Her remarks were cutting, stark. I am glad she was speaking in Telugu, otherwise, the clarity and force of her statement could have been lost in translation. In that moment, in concentric ways, she revealed how her life has been distilled to bear such burdens. This was her fate.

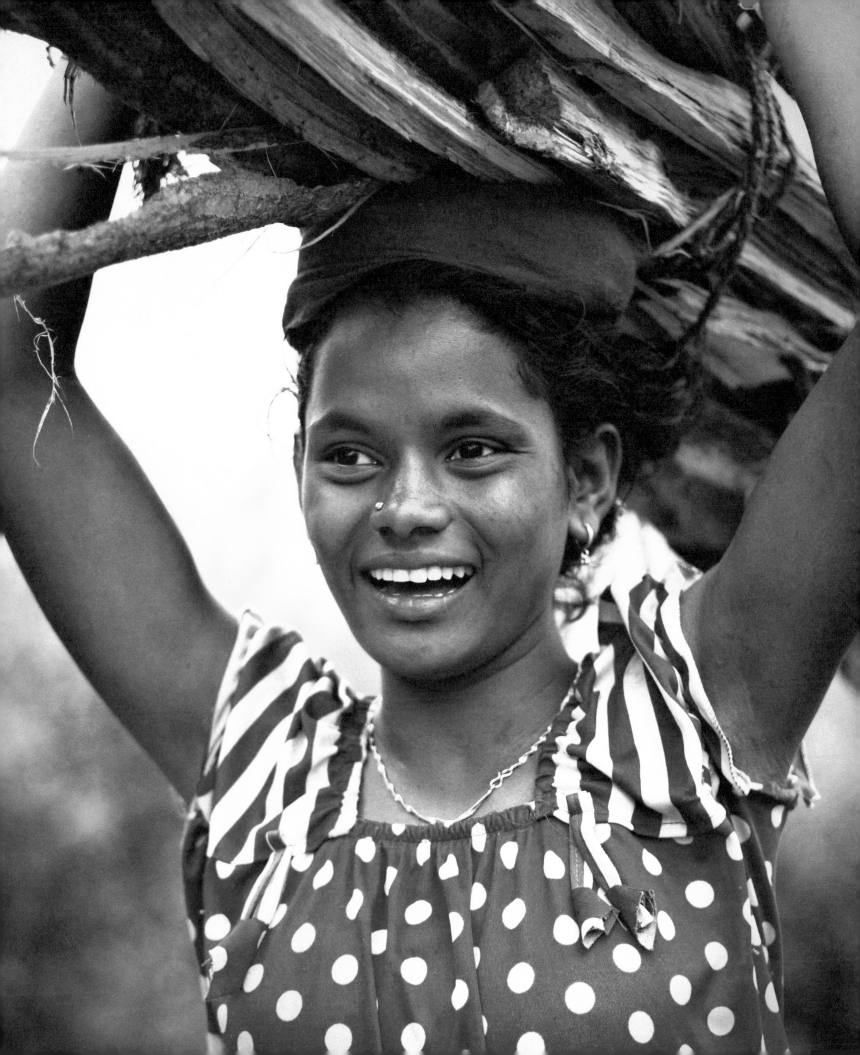

In part, this woman was admonishing me for asking my question, the answer to which was evident in the lives of the women standing in front of me. Her reply was a polite dressing-down, a minor protest of a difficult life she has not chosen, but to which she has resigned herself.

She endures the weight of a cultural expectation, compounded by household poverty, to shoulder a globally consequential burden: providing daily fuel for her household. Life for this woman, the others with her, and millions of others like them, is grueling. They pour out of jungles carrying firewood to heat their homes, to cook hot meals for their families.

This is the extraordinary daily story of 3 billion people primarily dependent on solid fuels to meet their daily household energy needs.[1] It is a complex story of poverty, culture, ecosystems, affordable technologies, environment, health, and gender inequalities that must be unpacked.

Without this daily hunt for fuel by millions of such women and children, there will be no fires in the hearth. Without these wood fires, there is no cooking and heating for billions around the globe. And yet: These everyday acts to secure household energy to sustain life produce large, irreversible, and tragic consequences for the health and productivity of people, their local ecosystems, and the environment. These acts are as essential as they are unsustainable.

BIOMASS AT THE CENTER
Biomass—in the form of fuelwood, agricultural residue, and animal waste—is among the most prevalent sources of energy in India, South Asia, and indeed throughout the developing world. The facts are bracing:

- While 3 billion people rely on solid fuels, 2.7 billion of these depend specifically on biomass energy for their daily cooking and heating; 1.3 billion are also without electricity; and 1.9 billion of them live in Asia, 84% of them in rural areas.[2]

- These 3 billion people burn a staggering 730 million tons of biomass at the rate of two tons by every family every year, and in aggregate 1 billion tons of carbon dioxide are released into the atmosphere.[3]

- Globally, cookstove smoke kills 4 million people a year—one person every eight seconds.[4]

- A recent World Energy Outlook report projects that by 2030, 2.7 billion people will continue to rely on biomass, with an estimated $1 trillion in cumulative investments needed to ensure modern energy access to these populations.[5]

- Narrowing our focus just to India, in that country alone 160 million households use solid fuels for heating and cooking, leading to 1,022,126 premature deaths annually.[6-9]

These numbers are numbing and unfathomable to most of us who do not directly experience energy poverty. These families are limited in their options for alternative fuels. Most are too poor to purchase household fuel in markets. Instead, they rely on tried-and-tested stoves: three stones with a pot on top and firewood underneath. However rudimentary, these stoves get families through the day, the week, the year. And as long as women and children are available—both physically and by prevailing social norms—to gather and hunt for firewood, a family is assured of daily fuel with which to cook and heat.

SOCIETAL NORMS
Why women and children? Culture and norms across South Asia and Sub-Saharan Africa dictate that they are responsible for gathering a household's wood, shrubs, dung, twigs, and other solid biomass for daily cooking and heating. They secure household energy from forest commons and other degraded common lands with shrubs and invasive species. Such degraded commons are mistakenly termed "wastelands," but in reality they are life-sustaining for a significant portion of the world's 3 billion energy poor.

When these commons don't exist, the burdens of women are multiplied. As forests and other commons decline or disappear, women and children are forced to walk greater distances to gather needed fuel for the family. Carrying heavier loads for longer distances comes at a cost to health, productivity, well-being, and life chances. Time spent collecting firewood is time away from tending to crops and other gainful tasks, as well as caring for children. For the children, it is time away from school.

1,210,193,422

2011 POPULATION

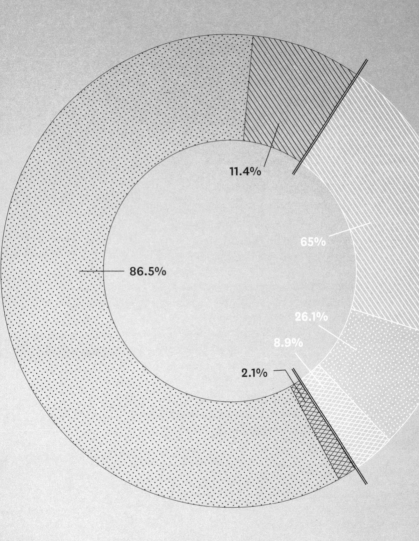

RURAL

68.84%

HOUSEHOLD ENERGY USAGE

 LPG/PNG

BIOMASS

OTHER

URBAN

31.16%

HOUSEHOLD ENERGY USAGE

LPG/PNG

BIOMASS

OTHER

11.4%

65%

86.5%

26.1%

8.9%

2.1%

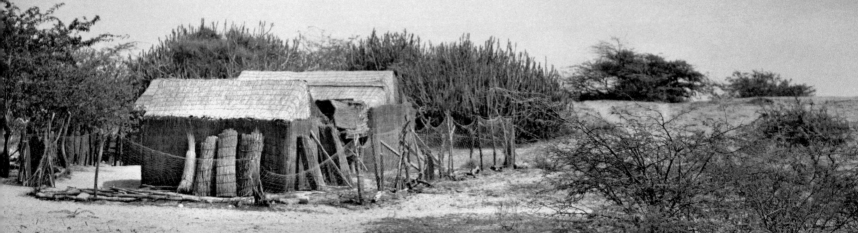

THE RIPPLE EFFECT

The ripple of impacts from gathering solid biomass extends not only to people, but to depleting groundwater systems, soil carbon release, and declining soil fertility, thereby leading to declining agricultural productivity, severely risking the future livelihood of these 3 billion. Such feedback accumulated in small acts of securing unclean solid biomass has massive and various impacts—from premature mortality and increased morbidity among these billions, to distressed local ecosystems, food insecurity due to low agricultural productivity, and eventually to a diminished future of another generation of several billion people. A cycle of interacting deprivations of energy, food, income, and water reinforces social, health, and educational deprivations among women and children. A cycle of hunting and burning fuelwood by billions converges, conspires, and corrodes these very lives over time.

Biomass combustion is also responsible for a significant proportion of carbonaceous aerosol emissions and "brown clouds" over the subcontinent.[11] Likewise, emissions from biomass combustion contain dangerous levels of fine particulate matter (PM2.5, PM10), carbon monoxide (CO), and nitrogen oxides, causing life-threatening and debilitating illnesses, especially in women and children.[12] Biomass combustion in millions of homes is a driver of increased infant and perinatal mortality; low birthweight; chronic bronchitis; chronic obstructive pulmonary disease; acute respiratory infections and decreased lung function; pulmonary tuberculosis; nasal pharyngeal, laryngeal, and lung cancer; adverse pregnancy outcomes; cataracts; ischemic heart disease; and cerebrovascular disease.[13-25] A staggering 4 million people die annually due to household air pollution from solid fuel combustion, and 99% of these deaths are in developing countries.[26] These damning health statistics are inevitable, when nearly 50% of the world's population is reliant on solid fuels for its everyday energy needs.

The World Health Organization accounts for the impact of such ill health on mortality and morbidity in a metric termed Disability Adjusted Life Year, or DALY. Each DALY is one lost year of healthy life, and when these years are summed across a population, they provide a snapshot of life lost due to disease. Put simply, the DALY is the disease burden on a society. In South Asia, 41.7 million life years are lost per year due to all forms of disease attributable to household air pollution from combusting solid fuels.

These cycles of interacting malignant processes are daily at play in India, which is home to 160 million households that rely on solid biomass to cook and heat.[27, 28] Even for an Indian economy experiencing a steady economic growth of 8% per year, it is difficult to spread the growth when two-thirds of the population is clean-energy poor, and thereby unproductive. Given the health, social, and economic externalities of being clean-energy poor, vast numbers of households are unable to engage in new opportunities that come from economic growth. No matter how rapid the economic growth, these 160 million households are a drag on sustainable development in India. Removing biomass from forests and in other lands changes the abundance and composition of woody species, threatening regeneration of ecosystems and livelihoods.[29] For these masses, a path toward sustainable energy systems—cleaner and more efficient—is a minefield of social, economic, and cultural preferences bounded by local ecosystems and risk-laden livelihoods that are ever-changing.

THE ROLE OF MENTAL MODELS

These preferences are further complicated by people's so-called "mental models," a term introduced by philosopher and psychologist Kenneth Craik to explain how we make sense of the external world. Craik's answer, as he put forth in his treatise *The Nature of Explanation* (1943), was this:

> Explanation, to the man in the street, means giving the causes of things and saying why they happen; and he is sure he perceives these external lasting things, though he may be mistaken about them on particular occasions.... [T]he final proof of anything must come from experience.[30]

In other words, mental models are therefore a representation of a possibility predicated on our experience.[31]

During my years spent in rural India, I have seen how mental models and available energy options shape household energy preferences and mold what is deemed practical and tenable. Here and throughout the world, mental models are also rooted in the social position an individual holds by virtue of his or her gender, class, caste, or household livelihood strategies; prior experiences borne out of a fixed social position; and knowledge of traditional and new energy systems, environmental quality, and local ecosystems. As Craik put it, "What is knowledge, if we are but a part of the mechanical system?"[32]

Individual and collective decisions flowing from these functional mental models over time accumulate to produce household energy preferences, resulting in changes in local ecosystems—which, in turn, shape future energy choices of rural households.

To many readers of this book, energy choices of the poor may seem puzzling, illogical, and self-defeating. But, in the words of the Princeton University professor Philip Johnson-Laird, a pioneer in the field of cognitive science, "Human reasoning is not simple, neat, and impeccable."[33]

Energy poverty is a complex story. It is a story of household poverty, and within it are multiple stories of women constrained by culture, of children—especially girls—sacrificed to meet daily household energy needs. It is a story of unsustainable lives, an unsustainable environment, and negative ecosystem outcomes. Untangling this Gordian knot to understand how several billion remain energy impoverished is not an easy undertaking, but we stand to gain insight into possible energy interventions that could prove effective and truly sustainable. These insights could be useful in designing technologies and interventions to tackle clean and efficient energy access for the many, providing sufficient quantity at a low cost. This is the energy challenge of our times.

GLOBAL ATTENTION AND ATTEMPTED INTERVENTIONS

Because of its massive scale and repercussions, the problem of rural household energy poverty has drawn global attention. The most notable effort thus far has been the Global Alliance for Clean Cookstoves, a partnership between academia, multilateral organizations, and the private sector. The Alliance was launched in 2010 at the Clinton Global Initiative with the goal of ensuring that 100 million households adopt efficient and clean cookstoves and fuels by the year 2020. The initiative is taking a market-based approach to catalyze the sector and ensure sustainable approaches and solutions in its promotion of clean cookstoves and fuels to save lives, improve livelihoods, empower women, and address adverse environmental impacts from using traditional stoves.[34]

The Global Alliance for Clean Cookstoves' ten-year strategic plan is a robust reboot to address adverse health and climate effects from the use of polluting cookstoves around the world. The Alliance's concern for understanding the use of cookstoves in the context of women's lives and their livelihoods marks a meaningful departure from previous cookstove efforts.

In addition, the Alliance is mounting a serious effort to understand barriers and enablers to cookstove uptake, in particular focusing on market enablers of cookstove dissemination and implementation. Toward this goal, the organization is studying ways to strengthen women as informed consumers of stoves, and develop markets that will provide multiple clean-cooking technology options and clean fuels.

Fundamental to the success of the Global Alliance for Clean Cookstoves will be sustained investments not just in public education and new technologies, but also in systematic transdisciplinary science—the call at the center of this book. Investments in science are needed for the development of cost-effective technologies that significantly reduce harmful health and environmental effects.

How clean is clean enough? Here, the goal should not be an imagined holy grail of cookstoves, but an array of "good enough" technologies that are perhaps 30, 40, or 50% more efficient than present-day cookstoves with successful uptake by a significant portion of those who are now combusting solid fuels. One recent study finds 90% more efficiency is needed to deliver positive health effects and meet WHO standards for household air quality.[35] Critical in this new approach will be transdisciplinary teams of practitioners, researchers, and consumers working together to produce new knowledge about technologies that are successful in rural households, sustainable in the way they are used, and affordable and available to these very communities.

Previous efforts at introducing efficient household energy systems have often failed because people are reluctant to use them, the new technology didn't perform in actual rural households (as opposed to an engineer's lab), or the new technology was used briefly but fell into disuse. Previous research on rural energy systems and household behavior has been distinctly disciplinary, framed exclusively by a single field, whether it is social science, engineering, or ecology.

Energy choices, however, are embedded in the logic of social norms, distressed ecosystems, and the daily living habits of people dependent on natural resources to supplement their livelihoods.

THE GLOBAL DEVASTATION OF HOUSEHOLD AIR POLLUTION [36]

UNPACKING THE DAMAGE

In India, household air pollution (HAP) from solid fuels is the third leading cause of death, killing 1 million people per year. But this grim statistic provides just a glimpse of the total scale of devastation attributable to HAP. Worldwide, the total deaths per year has reached 4 million, making HAP the fourth leading cause of death across the globe.

Women and children have greater exposure to household pollution and, as discussed in this book, disproportionately carry the burdens of securing household energy needs over men. Men, however, suffer more deaths from exposure to HAP: 2,577,672 deaths per year, compared to 1,611,730 for women. This is due to the inclusion of cardiovascular outcomes that increase the risk attributable to household smoke. While the *relative* burden for women from household air pollution is higher, the *absolute* burden is higher for men.

However, deaths do not give us the full picture of the burden of household air pollution on people. Disability Adjusted Life Years (DALYs, introduced on the previous spread) combine a metric for years of life lost due to premature

mortality in a population with years lost due to disability from incidence of a particular health condition. DALYs provide an aggregate measure of years of loss of healthy life in a country or a region, allowing us to envision the loss in people's productivity and contribution to society and the economy from incidence of a particular health condition. South Asia DALYs attributable to household air pollution are a staggering 41,728,844, compared to 2,538,754 for Latin America and the Caribbean. In South Asia, there are far more people experiencing loss in healthy life from exposure to household air pollution. Just for India, the latest estimates are 31,415,910 DALYs. Sub-Saharan Africa altogether registers 26,217,622 DALYs from exposure to household air pollution.

The challenge of household pollution is global, and India, with a large number of deaths and loss in healthy life, offers a generalizable case to explore solid fuels and their impact on people's health. The challenge is first to understand aerosol emissions from burning solid fuels in traditional stoves and then to design affordable, acceptable, and efficient energy systems.

DEATHS AND LOSS OF HEALTHY LIFE

FROM EXPOSURE TO HOUSEHOLD AIR POLLUTION

LATIN AMERICA & THE CARIBBEAN

DEATHS	DALYS
89,628	2,538,754

NORTH AFRICA & THE MIDDLE EAST

DEATHS	DALYS
25,683	921,904

SOUTH ASIA

DEATHS	DALYS
1,276,195	41,728,844

CENTRAL EUROPE, EASTERN EUROPE & CENTRAL ASIA

DEATHS	DALYS
161,387	3,521,008

SUB-SAHARAN AFRICA

DEATHS	DALYS
464,417	26,217,622

SOUTHEAST ASIA, EAST ASIA & OCEANIA

DEATHS	DALYS
1,460,717	33,117,896

UNDERSTANDING AEROSOL EMISSIONS

When many people hear the word "aerosols," they may think of a spray can of deodorant. This is not what we mean. An aerosol is defined as a system of solid or liquid particles suspended in air or other gaseous environments. Combustion systems promote this new particle formation. Fuel is combusted to create a high-temperature zone where heat is extracted and used for myriad applications, ranging from cooking food to generating power. The word "fire" is associated with all combustion systems—and plays a major role in the history of mankind.

While we think we have "controlled" fire, the formation of unwanted byproducts remains a concern—and we have not overcome those challenges. Fuels that are used (typically fossil fuels) have trace constituents that go through certain pathways and result in fine particle formation. Even in the best controlled systems that we use, we face challenges. The problem becomes even more acute when people in rural areas use fire to meet their cooking needs. They do not have access to well-designed and well-controlled combustors.

Ideally, a particular combustion system would oxidize all the carbonaceous species, and result in the formation of carbon dioxide, and maybe water vapor. This isn't happening, for two central reasons. One, the fuels that we use are not pure carbonaceous species, nor pure hydrocarbons that would result in formation of just carbon dioxide and water. And two, all engineered systems have thermodynamic and kinetic constraints; thus, it is practically impossible to have complete combustion that results in only carbon dioxide and water formation. For example, fossil fuels such as coal have a range of species such as trace metals that result in the formation of fine particles.

Fuels such as biomass also have species such as potassium, sodium, and other elements that go through the same pathway and form particles. More importantly, due to non-idealities in combustion, even the carbonaceous species are not completely oxidized and form a range of complex organic and carbonaceous species particles. In lay terms, we often call this "soot." The net is that any combustion system produces a high-number concentration of particles of varying compositions, and often these are problematic constituents that result in deleterious environmental and health effects.

Why are particles emitted from combustors so problematic? In short, they are part of a complex mix of particles, appearing in a range of shapes and sizes—most are small, in the submicrometer size ranges—and, once emitted, they have a long lifetime. Unlike raindrops in the atmosphere, they are not large enough to come crashing down to the surface of the earth. They merrily float around—and are carried long distances—until they eventually encounter a human. These ultrafine particles (less than 0.1 microns) have become a central focus to aerosol scientists.

When it comes to the rural poor using cookstoves with biomass, or other fuels that have just been gathered, the situation is even more dire. None of the industrial pollution-control systems are available. The stoves are not designed for effective combustion, let alone to minimize emissions. The particles formed do not even have to travel far—the mother cooking the meal, and the children playing around the mother, all get exposed to freshly formed particles.

—Pratim Biswas, Chairman and Lucy & Stanley Lopata Professor, Department of Energy, Environmental & Chemical Engineering, Washington University in St. Louis, and Director, McDonnell Academy Global Energy and Environmental Partnership

PARTICLE SIZE AND PATHWAYS

Particles created during combustion can be very small—in some cases 100 times smaller than the width (or thickness) of a human hair. The smaller these particles are, the deeper they are lodged in the lungs.

SIZE RANGES OF COMMONLY OCCURRING PARTICLES

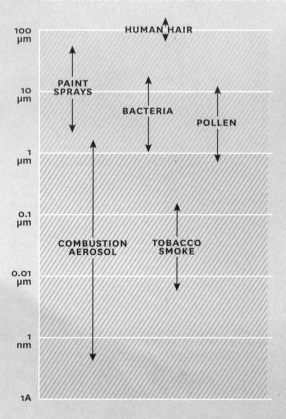

RESPIRATORY SYSTEM

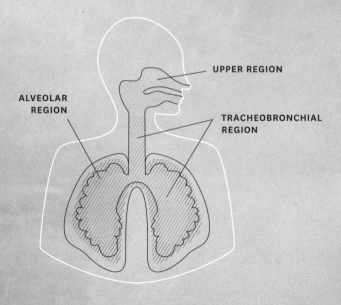

COMPARING VARIOUS COOKSTOVE EMISSIONS

Aerosol emissions from cookstoves are measured as particle mass concentrations, such as PM2.5—the total mass concentrations of all particles below 2.5 micrometers in size. In the figure at right, we chart the difference in the mass concentration of particulate matter measured close to the breathing zones of six cookstoves, from traditional to LPG. For comparison's sake, we have included the safe standards of PM2.5 according to the U.S. Environmental Protection Agency (EPA) and the World Health Organization (WHO), as well as where tobacco smoke falls on the scale. As you can see, even the most modern alternative stove remains dangerous for the user.

CONCENTRATIONS OF PARTICULATE MATTER (PM2.5) MEASURED CLOSE TO BREATHING ZONE WHEN USING VARIOUS COOKSTOVES[17]

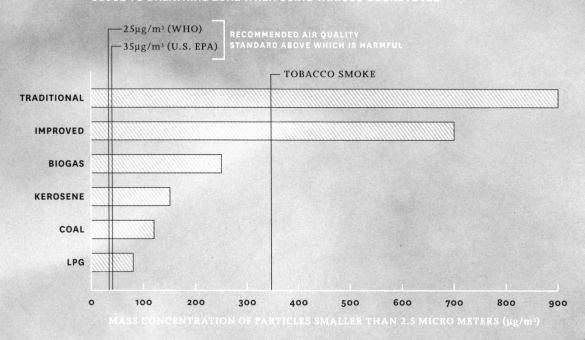

MASS CONCENTRATION OF PARTICLES SMALLER THAN 2.5 MICRO METERS (µg/m³)

EXAMINING THE SURFACE AREA OF PARTICLES

Beyond PM2.5, the Aerosol and Air Quality Research Laboratory at Washington University in St. Louis has measured the surface area concentration of particles deposited in the lung. This metric, measured for the first time for aerosols emitted from various cookstoves in rural areas in India, is shown in the figure at right. This data may be a more accurate representation of impacts on human health. While the particle mass concentration of emissions from a kerosene stove are relatively not high, the surface area concentration of particles deposited in the lung is very high. This is because the particles emitted from a kerosene stove are much smaller in size; and indeed, kerosene stoves are known to have more adverse health effects. This clearly illustrates the importance of using the correct metric for the evaluation of cookstoves.

SURFACE AREA CONCENTRATION OF PARTICLES DEPOSITING IN THE LUNG[20]

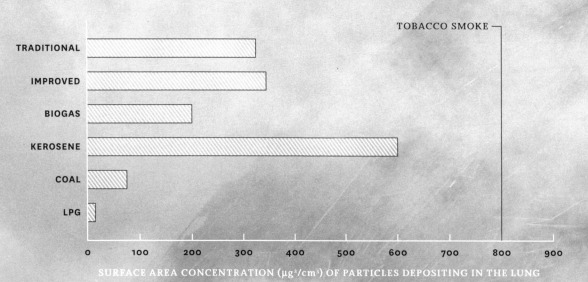

SURFACE AREA CONCENTRATION (µg²/cm³) OF PARTICLES DEPOSITING IN THE LUNG

LEAVING HOME

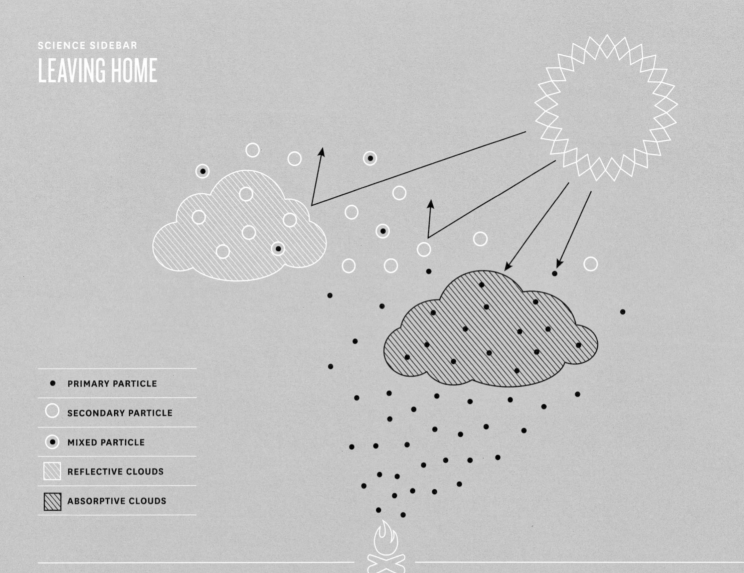

- ● PRIMARY PARTICLE
- ○ SECONDARY PARTICLE
- ◉ MIXED PARTICLE
- ▨ REFLECTIVE CLOUDS
- ▧ ABSORPTIVE CLOUDS

THE CONTINUED IMPACT OF AEROSOLS

Once these combustion particles (aerosols) and gases leave the home where they were produced, they continue to affect human health and go on to impact the global climate. Particles in the atmosphere have two general classifications:

1) **"Primary"** particles that are emitted directly to the atmosphere as particles; and

2) **"Secondary"** particles that were emitted as gases, but experienced sunlight-driven reactions to convert the gases into particles. Secondary particle mass can either form new particles or condense onto primary particles (making mixed primary/secondary particles). The ability to produce additional (secondary) particles in the atmosphere makes the combustion source even more relevant when viewing its impact regionally and even globally, since small particles can travel in the atmosphere for weeks.

Combustion sources can impact the climate in ways beyond the commonly discussed emission of greenhouse gases such as carbon dioxide, which act to warm the climate. Aerosols can directly impact our planet's energy balance by either absorbing sunlight (warming) or scattering sunlight (cooling), depending on the color of the particle. Aerosols can also indirectly affect the global energy balance by altering cloud formation, cloud reflectivity, and cloud lifetimes. Globally averaged, aerosols have a net cooling effect on the planet, countering (but not overpowering) the warming effect of greenhouse gases.

Most combustion sources, however, produce dark soot primary particles that have a warming effect on the climate. Little is known about the ability of combustion sources to produce secondary particles that could make some contribution toward cooling. Today, gaps remain in our understanding of how secondary particles are formed, and how primary and secondary particles directly and indirectly impact our climate. In fact, the main reason we don't know the exact extent to which humans have altered Earth's energy balance is due to our uncertainty of the direct and indirect aerosol effects on climate. This uncertainty brings additional challenges to accurately predicting climate trends, as we consider future changes to our energy production practices.[39]

—Brent Williams, Raymond R. Tucker Distinguished I-CARES Career Development Assistant Professor, Department of Energy, Environmental & Chemical Engineering, Washington University in St. Louis

Our challenge is to give prominence to understanding subtle and nuanced connections that link household energy choices, gender inequalities, ecologies, household emissions, impacts on environment, and the future abundance and composition of the forest ecosystem, an important source of fuelwood.

THE LIMITATIONS OF NEW TOOLS ALONE
To reduce the many negative effects of biomass combustion, governments and nongovernmental organizations (NGOs) throughout the developing world have undertaken interventions to disperse improved stoves that would require less fuel, reduce dangerous emissions, and yet meet the energy needs of rural households.

Although more efficient and emissions-reducing technologies can be produced in the laboratory, designing them to sustainably work in various sociocultural contexts has proved challenging. Improved stove-technology programs have often been unsuccessful because households do not adopt the improved technologies at all, or if they do adopt, use them in a way that does not achieve the sought-after level of reductions in fuelwood used and harmful emissions.[40, 41]

Hence, one of our challenges is to provide the poor with greater access to devices and fuels that can be sustainably used in a variety of real-world conditions. The more these are developed and tested in collaboration with these communities—particularly with the women, the devices' end users—the more likely their uptake. In seeking greater consistent uptake, we may also find that striving for, say, 90% or 100% efficiency is too big of a leap to make from where we stand today. Perhaps a technology that is only 40% more efficient might actually be twice as likely to be used consistently, because it is designed to be culturally compatible, meets the expectations of rural households (particularly women), and takes into account the type of wood available for burning. We then need to answer whether a 40% reduction in emissions will improve the health of women and children.

The failure of interventions so far stems from a surface understanding of household decision-making processes about fuel and efficient stoves. Household decisions have to be understood within the context of livelihoods of the rural poor: the social, political, cultural, economic, and ecological

dimensions of energy security, as well as access to alternative sources of energy and household strategies to meet fluctuating energy supply and demand.[42-44] We must accelerate our understanding of energy transitions, behavioral drivers of decisions to shift to newer efficient stoves, and the prevailing social and cultural norms that impact adoption and implementation of alternative energy technologies.[45]

A household's behavioral response to cleaner cooking technologies depends on its livelihood strategies, wealth, household composition, ecological quality, sustainable use and management of local natural resources, culture-based preferences around food preparation, and the time it takes to obtain traditional fuels.[46-49] A family's decision to adopt—or not to adopt—an improved cooking technology stems from how these factors influence a household's perception of the scarcity of traditional sources of energy (primarily fuelwood), as well as the actual scarcity. Where traditional fuels are not scarce, households are less likely to adopt new cooking technologies, and prefer to stay on the lower rungs of the energy ladder.[50-53]

THE ENERGY LADDER THEORY
Households transition from primitive to modern energy sources as they move up what is known as the "energy ladder." An energy ladder framework postulates that households prefer increasingly advanced forms of energy as their income rises, and in the process abandon traditional and primitive fuels for household energy.[54, 55]

While the energy ladder theory is intuitively appealing, it does not align with household behavior in rural India, South Asia, or Sub-Saharan Africa. Energy sources might not change dramatically with income among rural households, but as income rises, the aggregate demand for energy might still rise.[56] Moreover, households seldom transit in a linear fashion from primitive to modern sources of energy. There is considerable oscillation between types of energy sources, in large part due to the risk inherent in shifting from a tried-and-tested energy source to a newer fuel, combined with the uncertainty of income streams to maintain the more expensive and modern fuels.

Uncertainty in income is due to a host of factors, starting with rain-fed agriculture, a significant source of livelihood but at the mercy of increasing

KEROSENE IN FOCUS [57-62]

Kerosene is an important transitional fuel for lighting, cooking, and heating in homes that are reliant on solid fuels for household energy. Four to 25 billion liters of kerosene are used annually solely for lighting purposes; its use for cooking is also prevalent, though more so among urban households.

Only recently has kerosene gained attention for its negative environmental and health impacts. Kerosene lamps on their own emit 270,000 tonnes of black carbon into the atmosphere. The warming effect on the atmosphere from this black carbon is equal to 240 million tonnes of CO_2, a greenhouse gas. Eliminating current annual black carbon emissions is equivalent to reductions of 5 gigatons of carbon dioxide over the next twenty years.

Kerosene is also a cause for concern in women's and children's health, as it is associated with low birthweight and neonatal deaths. There is also an increased risk of stillbirths in households that use kerosene compared to cleaner fuels, even after controlling for other explanations. Reduction in kerosene use is possible through affordable LED lighting, combined with a rollback in subsidies for the fuel.

variability in rainfall. Income declines could be due to degraded ecosystems and declining soil fertility in the case of dryland communities experiencing decreasing levels of agriculture productivity.

A linear energy transition theory also glosses over a sizable segment of the 3 billion people that is on the move, knitting together a patchwork of livelihoods. This population might experience more income in migration. In their transient state, however, they resort to fuels that are easily available—wood, crop waste, woody shrubs, and other biomass that can be burned in a primitive stove. The other group on the move is pastoralists or herding populations that are transient, dispersed, and dependent on solid biomass in the midst of herding. Such transient groups are least likely to follow a linear path on the energy continuum and do not fit neatly into an energy ladder framework. Supplying this large group with a newly engineered stove simply would not create sustainable change.

Another reason why an energy ladder framework is not necessarily applicable is that many households don't always see fuelwood as inferior. In some cases—such as boiling water or preparing feed for livestock—fuelwood is better suited to the household task and clearly preferred over other superior fuels, even when income and access to modern fuels are nonissues.[63]

ENERGY STACKING

While the energy ladder theory has been influential in framing how the poor move along a continuum of fuels, always substituting traditional fuels with newer fuels, field studies and observations show that the poor are not on a linear path up the energy ladder.[64] Rural households, and even the urban poor, routinely use new sources of energy in tandem with more traditional fuels such as wood. Regular use of both old and new fuels by rural households poses a great challenge to exclusively promoting black carbon-reducing cookstoves.

A recent study of household energy use provides ample evidence for what has been termed "energy stacking" or "fuel stacking," where fuelwood use continues alongside electricity that is available and provided to all households.[65] This energy stacking is also evident when households are given new stove technologies, yet retain older, inefficient stoves alongside the newer devices, undermining the goals

of reducing black carbon emissions and improving the health of women and children.

Guarding against unexpected outcomes is somewhat common, and is akin to how many of us hold on to our cars even after a new metro train system is introduced, or save drawers full of paper copies of documents we are storing in "the cloud." Similarly, the drivers of energy stacking are too deeply entrenched in a household preference to avert risk, in the event that a new stove breaks down. This is understandable, given that typically households do not participate in the development of new stove technology and are only peripherally knowledgeable about the workings of that technology. Add to that all forms of risk that pervade their lives, and you can understand why it would be prudent to minimize risk, if possible.

The energy ladder framework also raises a more fundamental question of sustainability. Do we want the poor to move up this traditional energy ladder, passing through phases of coal, gas, natural gas, and electricity, and be on an unsustainable course that the rest of us have been climbing, only to contribute to greenhouse gases and a warming of the planet? Alternatively, do we want the poor to leapfrog to a new generation of low-carbon energy technologies that are clean and modern?

Moreover, households that repeatedly experience shocks to their livelihoods will naturally limit their risk (albeit at the margins), and not completely abandon reliable cookstoves for newer technology that they do not understand and have had no part in designing. The natural decision is to stack new technologies along with older technologies and in the process undermine any potential gains in the reduction of harmful emissions. The trajectory of poor households along the clean-energy continuum is not straightforward, as households do not move from one energy source to the next, leaving the former behind. This argument is further bolstered by the notion that fuelwood is not always deemed inferior, because, as mentioned earlier, it is better suited for some household uses, even if a family can afford more modern fuels.[66]

A CASE OF LPG

It is natural to assume that when a household shifts away from solid biomass, it moves to liquefied petroleum gas (LPG) for its superior and cleaner

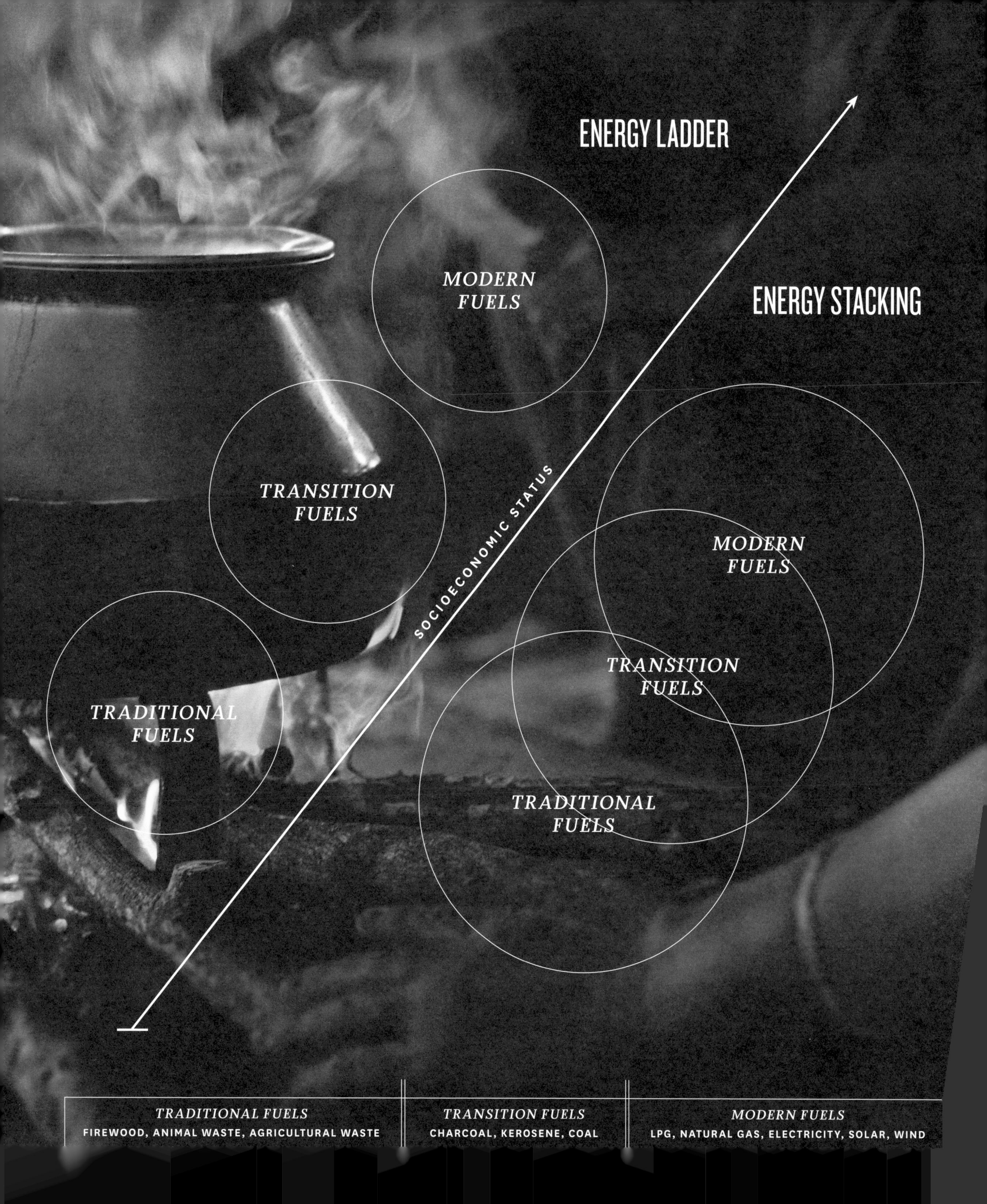

ENERGY LADDER

ENERGY STACKING

MODERN
FUELS

TRANSITION
FUELS

SOCIOECONOMIC STATUS

MODERN
FUELS

TRADITIONAL
FUELS

TRANSITION
FUELS

TRADITIONAL
FUELS

TRADITIONAL FUELS	TRANSITION FUELS	MODERN FUELS
FIREWOOD, ANIMAL WASTE, AGRICULTURAL WASTE	CHARCOAL, KEROSENE, COAL	LPG, NATURAL GAS, ELECTRICITY, SOLAR, WIND

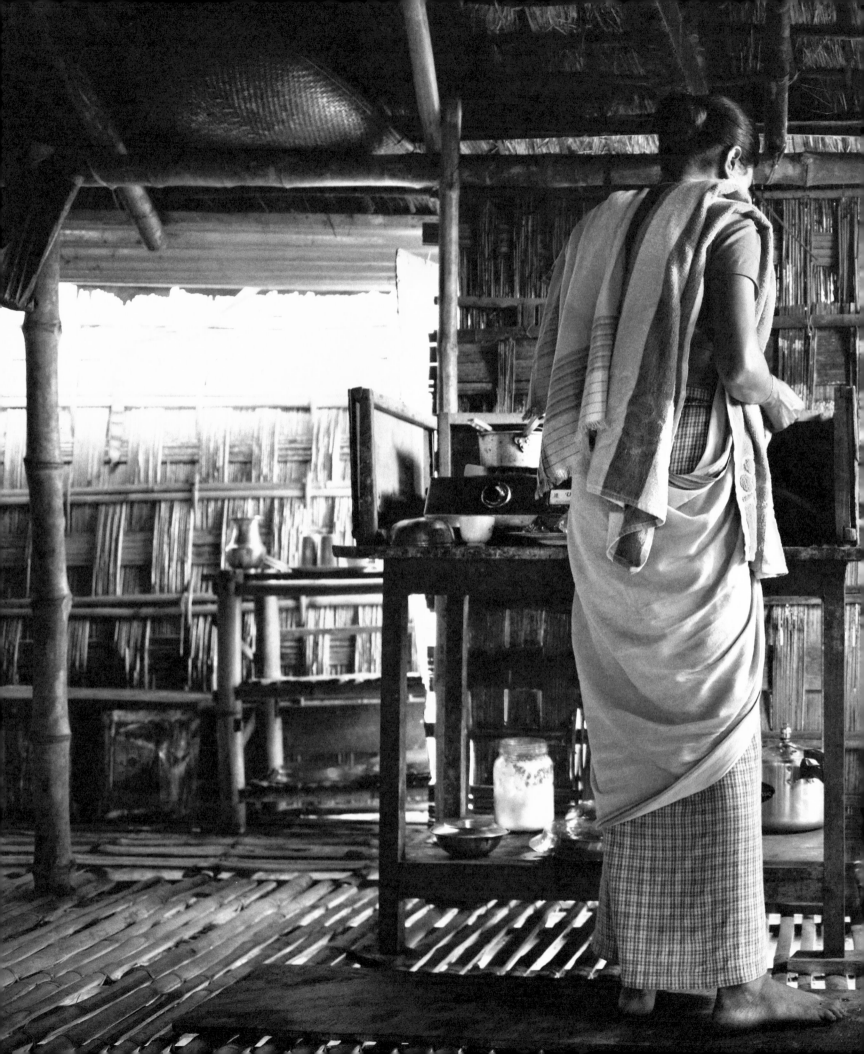

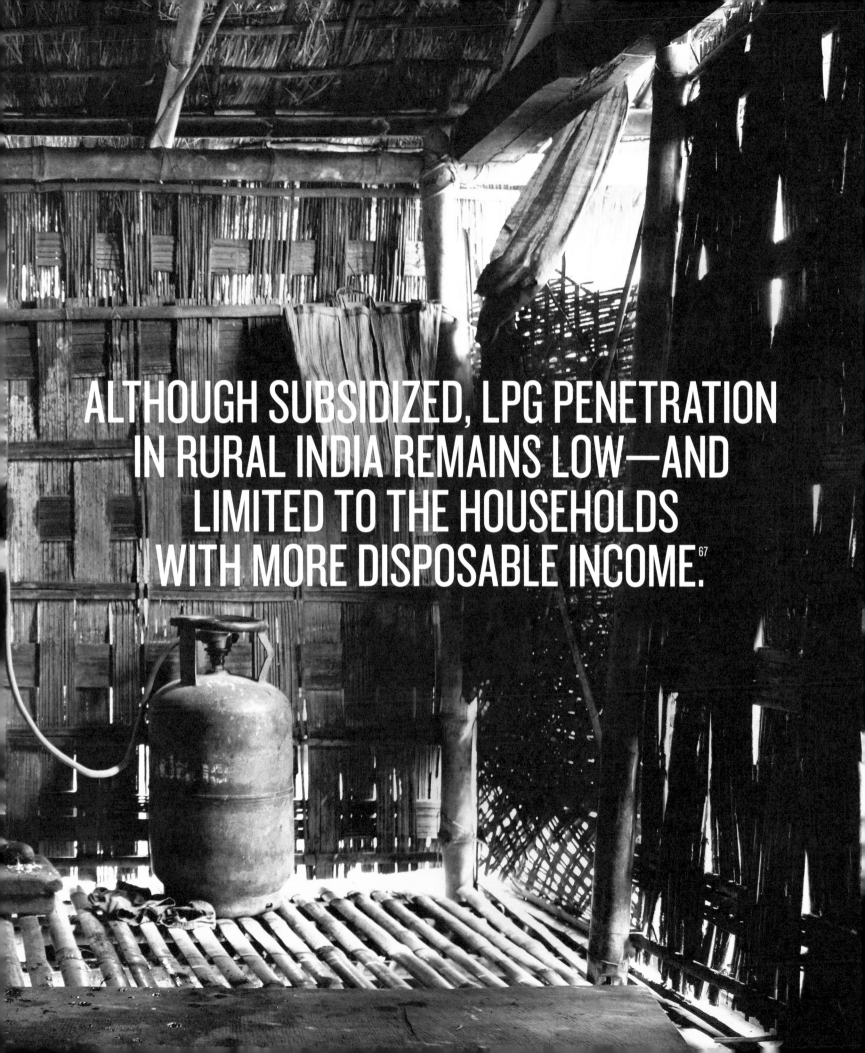

ALTHOUGH SUBSIDIZED, LPG PENETRATION IN RURAL INDIA REMAINS LOW—AND LIMITED TO THE HOUSEHOLDS WITH MORE DISPOSABLE INCOME.[67]

combustion. In a 2012 conversation I had with farmers in Anantapur district of Andhra Pradesh, I was impressed that in one village of 365 homes, some ten families had obtained LPG gas for cooking. As I spent more time discussing this shift by these ten households, to my surprise, their motivation was not to substitute LPG for solid biomass in traditional stoves. Yes, these families had more income and could afford to shift to cleaner cooking fuels. Instead, these well-off families told me they keep LPG for those times when extended family drops in unannounced. It is quick and easy to turn on an LPG stove and cook for more people than it is to begin stoking wood fires, which are smoky, inconvenience the guests, and take time to start. But for their own daily use, these families choose the traditional wood-burning stoves.

Far from moving to cleaner fuels, these families utilize LPG only for such emergencies. The farmers laughed at my assumption that these families would use it every day, especially when each cylinder costs 800 Indian rupees ($16 U.S. in winter 2012), and one has to travel at least fifty kilometers to the nearest crossroad town to obtain a cylinder. Remember that a mental model is an internal representation of a possibility. The farmers once again laughed at an assumption I made, this time that it is easier to obtain a cylinder of LPG than wood. For them, the possibility of easily obtaining wood is far greater. Consider this: for LPG they will have to go themselves to the nearest source fifty kilometers away, or hire someone to bring it from that far—compared to securing wood that women and children can obtain and carry back to the village. Even if wood is scarce, and may take more time to gather by women and children, these men were placing a premium on their own time away from the farm and the village, and simultaneously undervaluing the time it might take women and children to complete their task.

Compare these costs of obtaining LPG to gathering shrub and wood fuel that is available for collection within a few hours of walking by women and children who are "experts" at this—for whom it is "easy" to collect. That is the prerogative of men in a gender-unequal world, and my assumption that they would use clean cooking gas over wood is amusing, and even ridiculous, in their internal view of how the world works. To the men, wood is easier—but what about the women? Who prefers to

be an expert at carrying fifty kilos of wood, instead of switching to a lighter and cleaner fuel? The woman we met at this essay's beginning would say that women are meant to ensure what is needed for the household to cook, which is their fate, and therefore gathering wood is the easy and obvious decision to make.

Decisions about household energy and cooking technologies are subtle, complex, and nonlinear. Household decisions to adopt new technologies and alternative energy sources are motivated by factors endogenous and exogenous to the household, predicated on the technology itself, driven in part by the distressed state of local environments and biomass availability. Heterogeneous time preferences also are a factor in driving different classes of households to behave differently and invest in new technologies. Analysis of household dynamics of improved stoves will do well to heed time preferences, what economists refer to as discount rates—or time horizons—that the poor apply to their health and well-being, and account for household preferences for environmental outcomes.[68-72] The challenge of dissemination and implementation of new energy systems is to understand what drives short-term horizons and adaptive gender preferences, and overcome these and other individual and structural barriers to evidence-based interventions.

TWIN CHALLENGES OF DISSEMINATION AND IMPLEMENTATION OF NEW ENERGY SYSTEMS

How to interest communities and households in affordable and improved cookstoves shown to improve household air pollution, and what transpires after an improved, efficient cookstove has been provided to communities and households—these are the focus of dissemination and implementation. Over time, how will the implementer, the person whose behavior must change to take up the new cookstove, use it long enough to realize improved air quality and health benefits, even after the external supports have ceased?[73]

The assumption is that a cookstove deemed "improved" has passed a widely accepted standard for being efficacious and effective in more complete burning of biomass, with reduced levels of smoke and particulate matter. Clearly, we know the cause of poor health from burning biomass—dangerous smoke from burning wood in primitive stoves. This is called Type 1 evidence, where we have successfully defined the cause of the outcome. But we might still lack Type 2 evidence, which is evidence that a particular intervention, like an improved cookstove, actually reduces smoke and particulate matter that is the cause of the problem in the first place.[74]

The challenge of disseminating and implementing energy systems for the poor is to establish a greater degree of Type 2 evidence that improved cookstove interventions meet a certain standard of effectiveness to reduce household air pollution and improve health.

The other, more difficult challenge has to do with evidence that is needed for the adoption and implementation of new cookstoves—Type 3 evidence.[75] Under what conditions have improved cookstoves been successfully implemented, when do these improved stoves confront individual and structural barriers, and what evidence do we have to intervene to overcome such barriers?[76, 77] International efforts such as the Global Alliance for Clean Cookstoves have made both the development and promotion of international standards for improved cookstoves a priority area of work and a way to develop Type 3 evidence—knowledge that can lead to the effective dissemination and implementation of improved cookstoves across the globe under varied conditions.

Assuming that an improved stove meets a standard for being effective, the adoption and implementation of that stove are outcomes of household and individual decisions filtered through intrapersonal, interpersonal, and community traits. Successful implementation and sustainability of an improved stove are subject to the influence of informal opinion leaders, a woman's ability to exercise independent decisions within the household, the cost of the technology itself, and perceptions of the utility of an improved stove over a traditional stove, weighed against cultural predilections about abandoning old ways of cooking. Other structural factors have to do with the degree to which a household's decision to implement and sustain a new stove is driven by information and knowledge from outside the household or from external nonfamily and community organizations shown to be important in recent household energy research.[78] Nuanced evidence that provides insight into drivers that leverage successful implementation of new stoves is critical—and we can gather it when we rely

more on listening to communities, households, and people about their experience with new and old energy systems.

Let us remember my discussion with the farmers in the Anantapur district—even if some of them shift to cleaner stoves, they are still using them in combination with traditional stoves that burn solid biomass. This is the culture in that village. Cultural learning is in part responsible for adoption of new technologies and their use. There is mounting science that points to us humans as social learners who are far more focused on how others act; we learn from those actions.[79-80] Therefore, the role of community in shaping household preferences for clean-energy technologies and any shift in norms toward efficient combustion cannot be underestimated; increasingly, there is systematic research happening to understand how communities determine household decisions around fuel and combustion technologies.[82] The transition to clean energy and efficient combustion by the poor is possible only when the next generation of cleaner alternative fuels and efficient stoves are designed to be congruent with the dynamic complexity of community and household conditions and decisions.

Traditionally, disuse of a new stove technology has been quickly attributed to the social, economic, and cultural constraints that the rural poor face in the maintenance and use of a technology designed by outsiders. Another commonly proffered answer is that the stoves are incompatible with household practices, or that the poor have difficulties with the proper use and maintenance of new stove technology. The more important question we must answer is why the poor are unable to properly maintain technology that is deemed "superior," finding it incompatible with their lives.

We must answer these deeper questions before the next round of cleaner technologies are implemented and once more declared a failure in addressing harmful health and climate effects. Now that we are redoubling our efforts to promote efficient stoves to billions of poor in South Asia and Sub-Saharan Africa—through the Global Alliance for Clean Cookstoves Initiative, which will spend $50.8 million over the next five years, and other efforts from the Department of Energy and the U.S. Environmental Protection Agency—we cannot

ENERGY ACCESS AND MDGs[83]

Launched by the United Nations in 2000, the Millennium Development Goals (MDGs) aim to improve human well-being by reducing poverty, hunger, and child and maternal mortality, ensuring education for all, controlling and managing diseases, tackling gender disparity, ensuring sustainable development, and pursuing global partnerships. A key MDG is to reduce extreme poverty. Access to clean energy is critical to achieving this goal. Lack of access to clean energy undermines health and productivity, limits opportunities for education and development, and reduces a household's potential to rise out of poverty. Providing 1.9 billion people with sustainable access to modern fuels by 2015 would meet the Millennium Development Goal for poverty reduction.

A TRANSDISCIPLINARY APPROACH
TEAM SCIENCE FOR TEAM SOLUTIONS

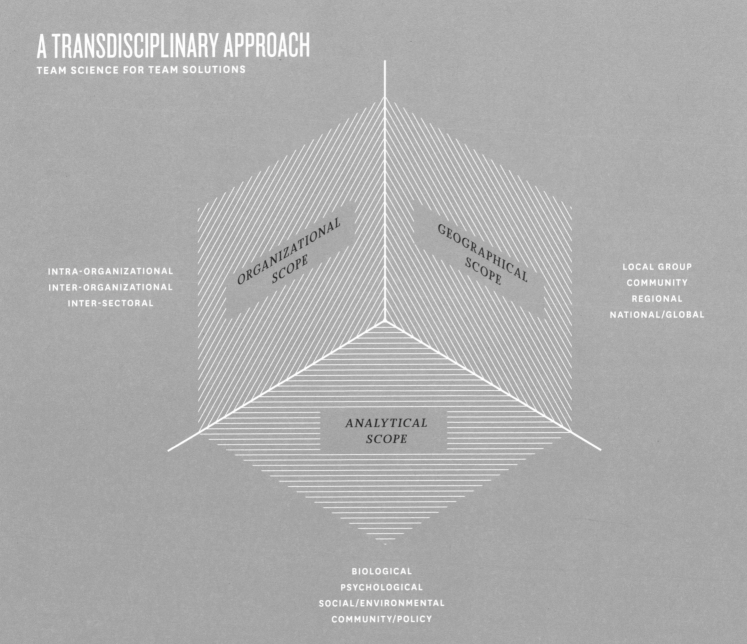

ORGANIZATIONAL SCOPE

GEOGRAPHICAL SCOPE

INTRA-ORGANIZATIONAL
INTER-ORGANIZATIONAL
INTER-SECTORAL

LOCAL GROUP
COMMUNITY
REGIONAL
NATIONAL/GLOBAL

ANALYTICAL SCOPE

BIOLOGICAL
PSYCHOLOGICAL
SOCIAL/ENVIRONMENTAL
COMMUNITY/POLICY

The problem of energy impoverishment sits at the intersection of a spectrum of disciplines. As such, it is a prime example of how even the most expert scientists can fail to solve a particular problem, as they haven't examined proximate, connected topics that emerge in other aspects of people's lives.

To tackle energy impoverishment, we must "undiscipline" ourselves, climb out from our academic silos to develop new conceptualizations of the problem—and only then build solutions that are both more likely to be taken up and more likely to scale successfully. Knowledge produced in isolation may serve specific actors but will not solve complex problems. A transdisciplinary approach emphasizes coproduction of knowledge and attempts to erode disciplinary barriers and the hierarchies between different ways of knowledge production: traditional vs. scientific.[84]

The above figure, adapted from work by the University of California–Irvine's Daniel Stokols,[85] illustrates the demands of transdisciplinary research, the need to expand the analytic, organizational, and geographic scope to address complex and dynamic problems like the uptake and sustained use of clean-energy systems by the energy poor.

Organizations must transition from working just among themselves to working with similar organizations (two universities, for example), to working with groups from entirely different sectors (with governmental and non-governmental agencies joining in as well).

Our analytical lens must encompass many disciplines—from biology and ecology to engineering, behavioral economics, and other social sciences.

Geographically, current research on the energy poor is being done at a particular scale of hamlets, villages, districts, and regions. But the livelihoods of households that depend on biomass fuels are not confined to small geographies. Teams must work at multiple scales—from local groups to regional to national to global.

afford to remain satisfied with answers at a certain generality. We must probe deeper into both the household and larger drivers of uptake of sustainable new technologies in rural societies. We must demand systematic answers to effectively redress previous failures and give emphasis to mental models of the poor, and give prominence to their worldviews, amplifying their voices and preferences in our efforts at designing and promoting clean and efficient energy technologies.

INTEGRATING SYSTEMS SCIENCE INTO DISSEMINATION AND IMPLEMENTATION

What distinguishes those who successfully adopt and implement an improved cookstove from others who abandon it in just a short period? Could the root cause of success or failure in implementation be the intervention itself—the new cookstove? Does the explanation lie with structural and relational drivers that differentiate those who take up, successfully implement, and sustain innovations over time to realize substantial gains in health? Generating systematic evidence to these questions about improved cookstoves will improve what has been described in dissemination and implementation science as the "external validity of interventions, the replication of positive effects across dissimilar settings and conditions, and scale-up, the replication of positive effects across similar settings and conditions."[86]

For this, we need a greater emphasis on systems science in cookstove dissemination and implementation to disentangle and understand with greater clarity the emergent nature of human behavior, social norms, the nature of gendered relations, and the use and performance of cookstove innovations, all in the context of community, and local ecosystems—storehouses of biomass used in cooking. The use of systems science methods in the dissemination and implementation of new cookstoves and other alternative energy systems is at an early stage. Public health experts have declared dissemination and implementation to be a complex and dynamic social and organizational process, and have turned to systems thinking and systems science for deeper insights on the processes that drive diffusion of innovations, and factors that differentiate early adopters from late adopters.[87]

Systems analysis of dissemination of clean cookstoves and other clean-energy technologies has to be done on the ground, where such interactions are unfolding and influencing the sustainability of these new interventions. Communities and people become the central focus. Systems thinking reorients dissemination and implementation, and privileges a more practice-based evidence, where learning is happening about how different subsystems are interconnected in a structure of feedback mechanisms.[88] Community, people, households, their worldview, and their motivation for actions now become central in the science of understanding implementation of innovations.

Assuming that we have overcome our first challenge—that the intervention meets a certain standard of improvement over current cookstove technologies—the major remaining challenge is to deploy these new technologies successfully. In this challenge, collaboration with communities and households is paramount, and their participation in the dissemination and implementation of new cookstoves and alternative energy systems is essential.

PURSUING COLLABORATION AND PARTICIPATION

How does one listen and collaborate with the poor, particularly women, to produce clean and complete-combusting stove technologies and not dictate "appropriate" technologies? Participation in development programs is a promise of inclusion. Fully inclusive participation is a way to shift the axis of power and enable new actors to gain greater influence on outcomes related to their development and human condition. It is a path away from the language of target groups and beneficiaries, and toward citizenship, agency, governance, and rights.[89-91] When participatory processes tend to emphasize consensus, even well-intentioned participatory institutions can exacerbate existing forms of exclusion, silencing dissidence, and masking dissent. Indeed, the voices of the more marginal may not even be raised in such institutional spaces, thereby undermining the project of inclusion in social and economic development. Women's marginalization and that of the very poor is not one-dimensional—i.e., it is not caused only by gender or only by poverty. Rather, it is an outcome of the intersection of multiple forms of subordination, especially so in Indian villages, which are highly stratified by caste, class, ethnicity, and gender.

So how does one give serious consideration to the poor, and collaborate to obtain and share knowledge toward the common purpose of designing effective technologies to mitigate black carbon emissions from biomass combustion? Perhaps equitable collaboration across disciplines and stakeholders in different informational spaces will lead to effective clean-energy technologies with sustained uptake by the poor.

We must build respectful trading zones of knowledge among the users and designers of modern energy systems that will result in shared mental models of the problem at hand, instead of imposing predetermined solutions on the poor.[92] If efficient stove technologies and clean fuels are to make a difference in the lives of the poor, and for the climate, then we must create research paradigms reflecting a deeper understanding of the societal dimensions that are shared by the poor experiencing harmful household emissions—engineers working on combustion and aerosols; and social scientists working at the intersections of environment and development.[93] A consequence of such shared mental models is a moral imagination that transcends multidisciplinary collaboration to reach what Daniel Stokols and his colleagues have called "true transdisciplinary collaboration."[94] The tendency for certain stakeholders to dominate in the process of innovation has been the history of previous improved stove efforts.

Kirk Smith, a leading researcher and voice for intervening in health and environmental outcomes of solid fuel combustion, classifies the history of improved stoves into various phases—first focusing on smoke exposure, then on improving fuel efficiency, then moving on to a "phoenix phase" that combines the experiences of past failures (though even this phase fails to consider the context, local circumstances, and priorities).[95] Smith's lament is that outsiders have traditionally determined what is required, and steered the next phase in the innovation of efficient stove technologies. Successful models of transdisciplinary work can be transformative in affecting real-world problems, but also in changing the worldview of engineers and social scientists alike. Only in creating citizen scientists with deep public engagement and an awareness of the dynamic processes of biomass-dependent poor will we be able to arrive at a point of doing things differently.[96]

A "WICKED PROBLEM"

Writing in *Policy Sciences* nearly four decades ago, professors Horst Rittel and Melvin Webber reflected on how well-intentioned, careful planning built on the notions of efficiency had been futile in addressing societal problems.[97] The problems of scientists and engineers, they wrote, were tame and benign when compared to malignant, vicious, aggressive, and tricky societal problems. They termed these "wicked problems."[98]

Moving 160 million households in India to forgo primitive stoves and use cleaner fuels and cleaner-combusting stoves has all the makings of a wicked problem:

- The problem is difficult to formulate, as the definition is predicated on one's idea of how to solve it.

- There are no set criteria to know when we have solved the problem perfectly. We have only "good enough" solutions at best.

- Acceptable solutions are not clean dichotomies between true and false, but better or worse, or good enough.

- The problem of concern could itself be a symptom of another problem.

- Explanations and causal attributions of the problem are numerous, from that of a professional to those embedded in the problem.[99]

The problem of energy impoverishment feels like a moving target, with feedback effects that reinforce the dependence of the energy poor on biomass fuels, deforesting and degrading ecosystems, eroding health due to household air pollution, reducing productivity of women and the next generation of children, and further eroding ecosystems and soil fertility, reducing agriculture productivity, and increasing food insecurity. Cyclical relationships, a defining characteristic of wicked problems, are bound to have feedback effects from attempted interventions.

At the core of this problem are the realities of declining water, increasing air pollution, deforestation and ecosystem degradation, and climate impacts, forcing the chronically poor to make choices with significant implications for both the environment and their own future well-being.

Remember the young woman helping her sister carry fuelwood out of the forest in Orissa? Her real preference, it is obvious to us all, is not to carry that heavy load for several hours that day. She chose that, but it does not mean she prefers it to staying at home and relaxing with her sister.

Nobel laureate Amartya Sen, as well as the distinguished philosopher Martha C. Nussbaum, have deeply studied the lives women live, and ruminated on the pathways out of deprivation and poverty. Both Sen and Nussbaum have given serious attention to understanding the plight of the deprived and the perils of putting too much emphasis on the decisions people make under adverse circumstances. In his important 1999 book *Development as Freedom*, Sen wrote:

> Our desires and pleasure-taking abilities adjust to circumstances, especially to make life bearable in adverse situations. The utility calculus can be deeply unfair to those who are persistently deprived: for example, the usual underdogs in stratified societies, perennially oppressed minorities in intolerant communities, traditionally precarious sharecroppers living in a world of uncertainty, routinely overworked sweatshop employees in exploitative economic arrangements, hopelessly subdued housewives in severely sexist cultures. The deprived people tend to come to terms with their deprivation because of the sheer necessity of survival, and they may, as a result, lack the courage to demand any radical change, may even adjust their desires and expectations to what they unambitiously see as feasible... These considerations require a broader informational base, focusing particularly on people's capability to choose the lives they have reason to value.[100]

Sen is concerned about our tendency to be satisfied and accept the preferences and choices women make, as if they are their real preferences. Women make choices within a culture that obliges them to collect firewood for several hours, rather than one that would compel their families to adopt alternative energy solutions.

Nussbaum, in *Women and Human Development: The Capabilities Approach* (2000), traces the pernicious consequence of such adaptive preferences of women. Desires adjusting to one's way of life—adaptive preferences—are borne out of oppression and deprivation. They are distorted preferences. "Adaptive preferences," Nussbaum wrote, "are formed without one's control or awareness, by a causal mechanism that isn't of one's own choosing."[101]

Masking these adaptive preferences is the preferred choice of these women; Nussbaum would say that the challenge is to focus on the capabilities of these women so they make their preferred decisions over adaptive preferences. For this to happen, women have to "go through a two-stage process of awareness: coming to see themselves as in a bad situation, and coming to see themselves as citizens who had a right to a better situation."[102]

REINFORCING FEEDBACK

The underlying mechanisms that link household energy choices, rural livelihoods, and local ecosystems are complex and structured in an intricate web of what is known in systems science as "feedback mechanisms." These feedback mechanisms and processes among different types of fuel and combustion (biomass from native and invasive species, or cleaner fuels, and traditional to efficient combustion) and the impact on local forest ecosystem structure are subtle, accumulating, and dynamic over time. Central to these mechanisms are not only the biophysical properties of forests and local ecosystems providing biomass for household energy, but also human intervention and behavior. These vary depending on the livelihood strategies of a population, and the local ecosystems that are central to such livelihoods. The feedback mechanisms differ by the type of landscape—dryland agricultural regions, to river systems, to grasslands, or forests. Dynamic behavior between human, ecological, and energy systems is produced by multiple interacting feedback mechanisms. Some of these mechanisms are represented in a causal loop diagram on the following spread that unpacks some of the ways in which energy, environment, and poverty are bound together.

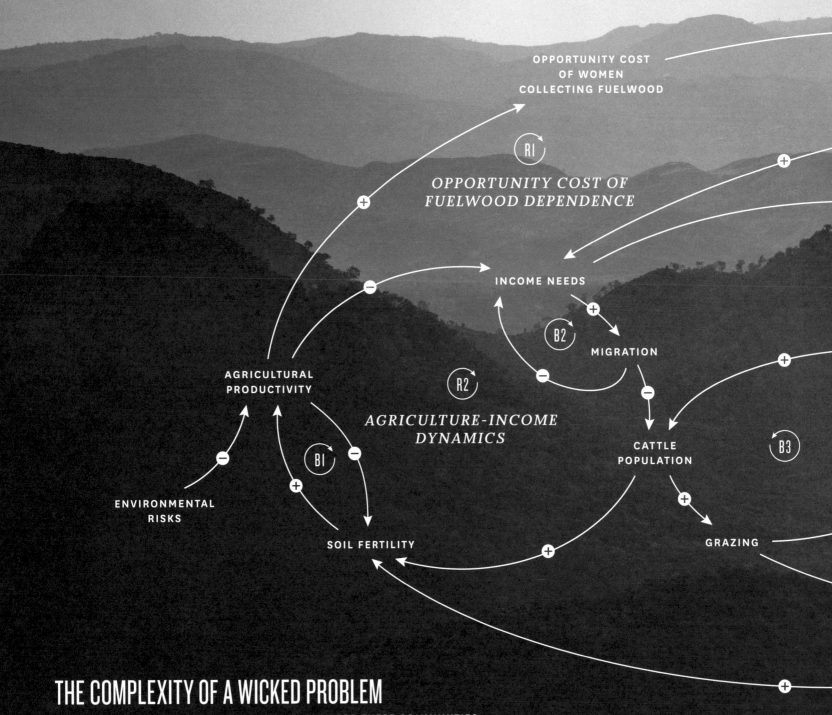

OPPORTUNITY COST
OF WOMEN
COLLECTING FUELWOOD

R1

OPPORTUNITY COST OF
FUELWOOD DEPENDENCE

+

INCOME NEEDS

+

B2

MIGRATION

AGRICULTURAL
PRODUCTIVITY

–

R2

AGRICULTURE-INCOME
DYNAMICS

–

CATTLE
POPULATION

B3

B1

–

ENVIRONMENTAL
RISKS

–

+

+

SOIL FERTILITY

+

GRAZING

+

THE COMPLEXITY OF A WICKED PROBLEM

EXPLORING THE FEEDBACK MECHANISMS IN PLAY FOR THESE COMMUNITIES

Navigating This Causal Map
*Efficient stoves, solar panels, and biogas stoves
all exist within larger systems. We might start with
a keen focus on the stove, but quickly come up
against other systems that either propel or impede
the stove's uptake. A careful navigation of the
causal map on this spread should provide a sense
of the other systems that are equally important in
understanding the use of clean energy by the poor.
This general causal map synthesizes a number of
insights about the use of clean energy technologies
by rural communities and how adjacent social,
agriculture, forest, and animal husbandry systems*

*from multiple conversations with a variety of
communities in Andhra Pradesh. It provides a
ground-level perspective of how communities
perceive energy systems and the influence of
other systems.*

Opportunity Cost of Fuelwood Dependence (R1)
When agricultural livelihoods are tenuous, as they
are in drylands of Andhra Pradesh or Rajasthan,
there is a decline in the opportunity cost of
deploying time and labor in other income-earning
household maintenance activities away from
agriculture. This loop illustrates the reinforcing
nature of fragile agricultural systems that

increase dependence on fuelwood for income
and household energy. With such transitions,
loss in forest diversity—in tandem with a decline
in uptake of any alternative clean-energy systems
in lieu of traditional wood-burning stoves—
amounts in time to adverse health outcomes.
Eventually, adverse health translates to declining
productivity. Over time, via other ecosystem
function mechanisms, forest diversity affects
agricultural productivity.

Agriculture-Income Dynamics (R2)
Outmigration of younger populations from villages
is predicated on income shocks due to variable

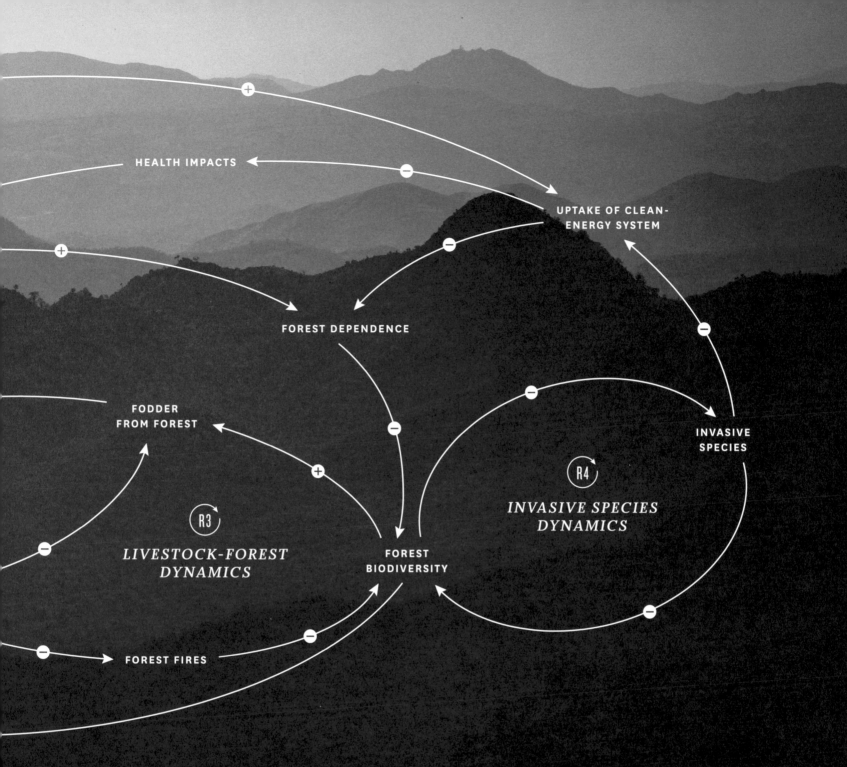

HEALTH IMPACTS

UPTAKE OF CLEAN-ENERGY SYSTEM

FOREST DEPENDENCE

FODDER FROM FOREST

INVASIVE SPECIES

R3

LIVESTOCK-FOREST DYNAMICS

R4

INVASIVE SPECIES DYNAMICS

FOREST BIODIVERSITY

FOREST FIRES

agricultural productivity. This productivity is highly variable when there are declines in soil fertility, an increase in exogenous environmental risks such as droughts, pestilence, and floods. In part, a decline in soil fertility is endogenous to cattle holdings, because as cattle holdings decline, the aggregate available organic manure also falls.

Livestock-Forest Dynamics (R3)
Demographic transitions in people and cattle holdings through time affect grazing practices in forests, creating a higher or lower propensity for forest damage through fires; in turn, these fires affect forest biodiversity with implications for

fodder production from forests to maintain a level of cattle holdings. Cattle holdings themselves are an outcome of migration from rural to urban and peri-urban areas.

Invasive Species Dynamics (R4)
Sustained forest biodiversity over time helps in the maintenance of ecosystem functions such as nutrient recycling, production of organic matter, and the release and capture of nutrients. Greater forest biodiversity also maintains ecosystem services at a high level, where food, water, and fuelwood are more abundant. Biodiversity is also critical for resisting invasive plant species, and

plant diversity increases carbon sequestration, nutrient richness, and soil organic matter. Here, we are focusing particularly on how forest biodiversity through time regulates the growth of invasive species and has reinforcing feedback in increased forest biodiversity.

Balancing Loops (B1, B2, and B3)
In a balancing loop, an action produces changes in the present situation to attain a desired situation. In B2, need for income causes migration. Migration lessens income need, which over time reduces the need to migrate.

SYSTEMS THINKING[103]

"Systems thinking is the mental effort to uncover endogenous sources of system behavior."

GEORGE P. RICHARDSON
System Dynamicist

The figure on the previous spread, while serving a heuristic purpose, shows some of the reinforcing feedback mechanisms that might be at play for the communities you will meet in this book. Sustained forest biodiversity over time helps in the maintenance of ecosystem functions, such as nutrient recycling, production of organic matter, and the release and capture of nutrients. Greater forest biodiversity also maintains ecosystem services at a high level, where food, water, and fuelwood are more abundant. Forest biodiversity is also critical for resisting invasive plant species, and with diversity in plants, there is greater carbon sequestration, nutrient richness, and soil organic matter, helping sustain forest biodiversity through time. Forest biodiversity and animal husbandry of farming households are interlinked through fodder production to maintain strong holdings of cattle. Organic manure from cattle and nutrient-rich runoff from biodiverse forests affect the soil fertility of farmlands and, through time, the agricultural productivity and income streams of households. These varied driving forces influence the extent of forest dependence in communities to supplement income and other household necessities, particularly energy needs. Environmental perturbations could decrease agricultural productivity and lower the opportunity costs of deploying household labor to collect fuelwood and engage in other income-generating activities. Increased dependence on free fuelwood could very likely increase the cost of migrating to more efficient and cleaner energy systems, further consolidating traditional stoves and fuels with adverse consequences for human health and environmental systems.

This conceptual model underscores for the reader how mental models of the sustainability of certain fuels reinforce the use of traditional biomass and combustion practices over cleaner fuels and efficient combustion, and through time cause significant shifts in forest ecosystems, agro-pastoral systems, and crop and livestock productivity, which in turn influence household energy choices.

To illustrate, let us posit that the shared experience of women and girls in rural India with the primary responsibility to collect biomass fuel drives them to adapt to easily available invasive plant species as fuel, thus driving changes in forest ecosystems and shifts in community incentives to manage invasive species. This leads to the establishment of new fire and soil fertility regimes, which in turn increase the rate of growth of invasive species relative to native species, and over time, plant biomass from invasive species becomes the dominant household fuel in a community. While households may successfully adapt in shifting to biomass fuel derived from an invasive plant species, the long-term impacts on forest biodiversity, household air quality, human health, and rural livelihoods remain unclear. To truly initiate the sustainable use of efficient stoves and clean fuels, we must disentangle these dynamic shifts over time in order to understand the co-occurring pathways of household energy choices, ecosystem structure and function, and rural livelihoods.

Providing access to clean, cost-effective energy systems for the poor is clearly a complex undertaking. When we hyper-focus on clean-energy systems, we lose perspective of the larger systems in which these interventions are deployed, including livelihoods dependent on rain-fed agriculture in semi-arid environments that can be drought-prone. In exclusively focusing on clean-energy technologies, we ignore dynamically complex systems in which we are introducing these innovations and fail in our dissemination and implementation. In pulling back the lens, we gain a better understanding of the interacting social, economic, cultural, natural resource, and market forces on people's lives that form the backdrop for these innovations.

The energy poor are embedded in dynamic systems that are changing over time, and behaviors emerge from an underlying mechanism of feedback structures.[104] For clean-energy systems to be taken up by the vast swath of the poor, we have to understand that translating efficacious interventions is not a one-off exercise. To disseminate and implement new energy systems, we must reframe the relevant boundaries; we must recognize the limits imposed by gender inequalities, or by the poverty and vulnerability of households on the uptake of new stoves. Household decisions about clean-energy systems are an outcome of interactions among household decision-making, livelihood practices, and landscapes in which livelihoods are embedded, and the vulnerability of households to shocks and stresses. It is time we shifted our focus to the households themselves. ✦

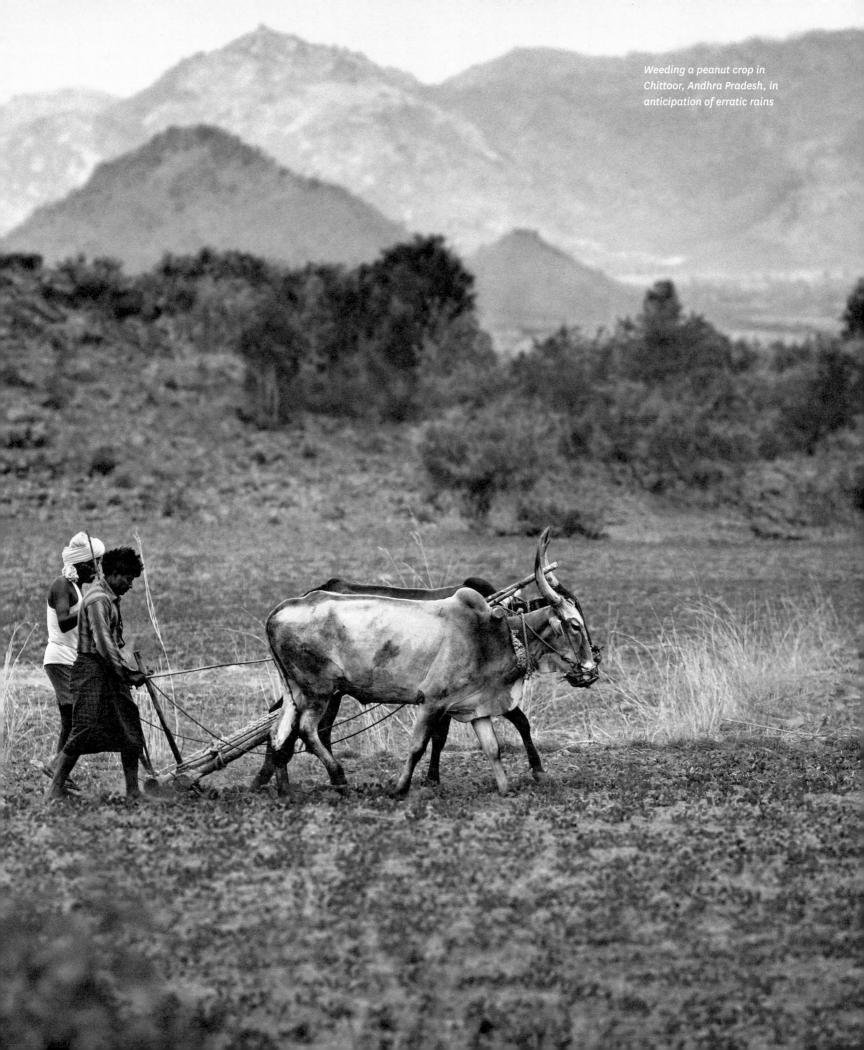

Weeding a peanut crop in Chittoor, Andhra Pradesh, in anticipation of erratic rains

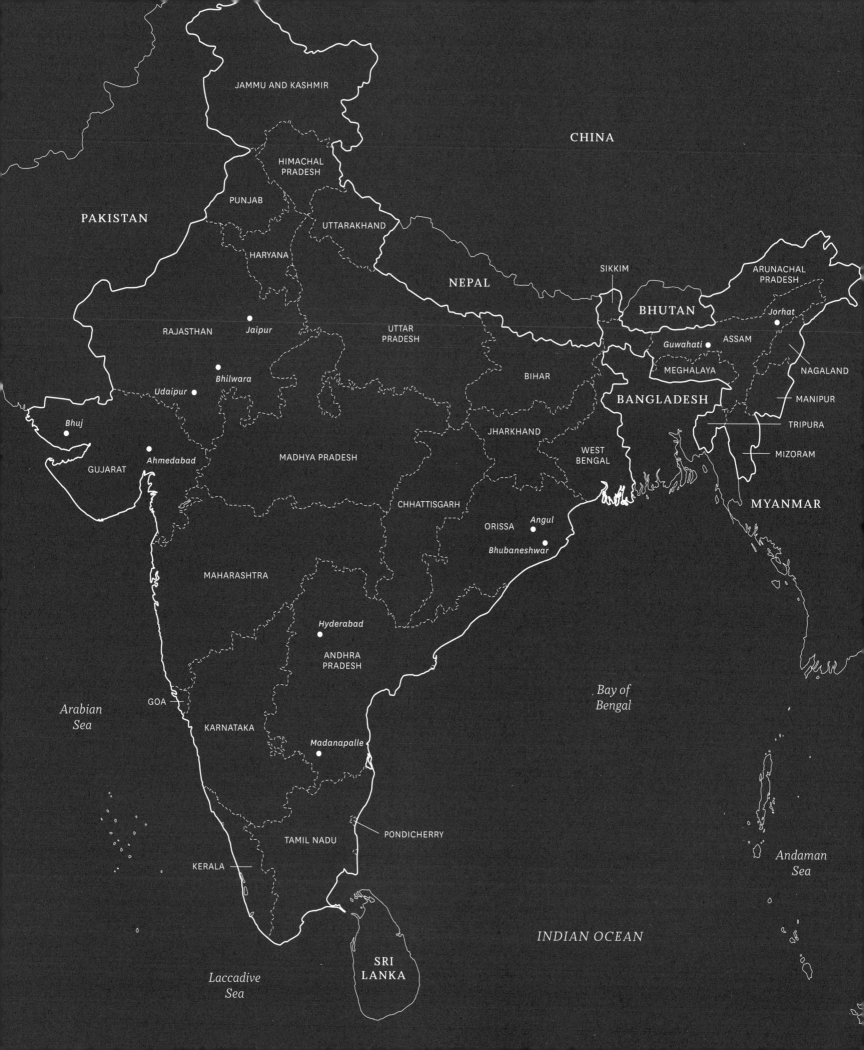

To best convey the critical task of providing billions of people access to clean-energy systems, we must explore the lives of a few to understand the myriad daily forces that shape the lives of the many.

Their ecosystems, cultural practices, agro-pastoral systems, and notions of viable livelihood strategies drive energy systems and decisions, whether these people live in marginal desert environments, river systems, or drylands.

In the following five stories, you will get a sense of the fragility of the energy impoverished, their reasoning for household energy decisions, and their tenacity and resilience in adapting to changing livelihoods.

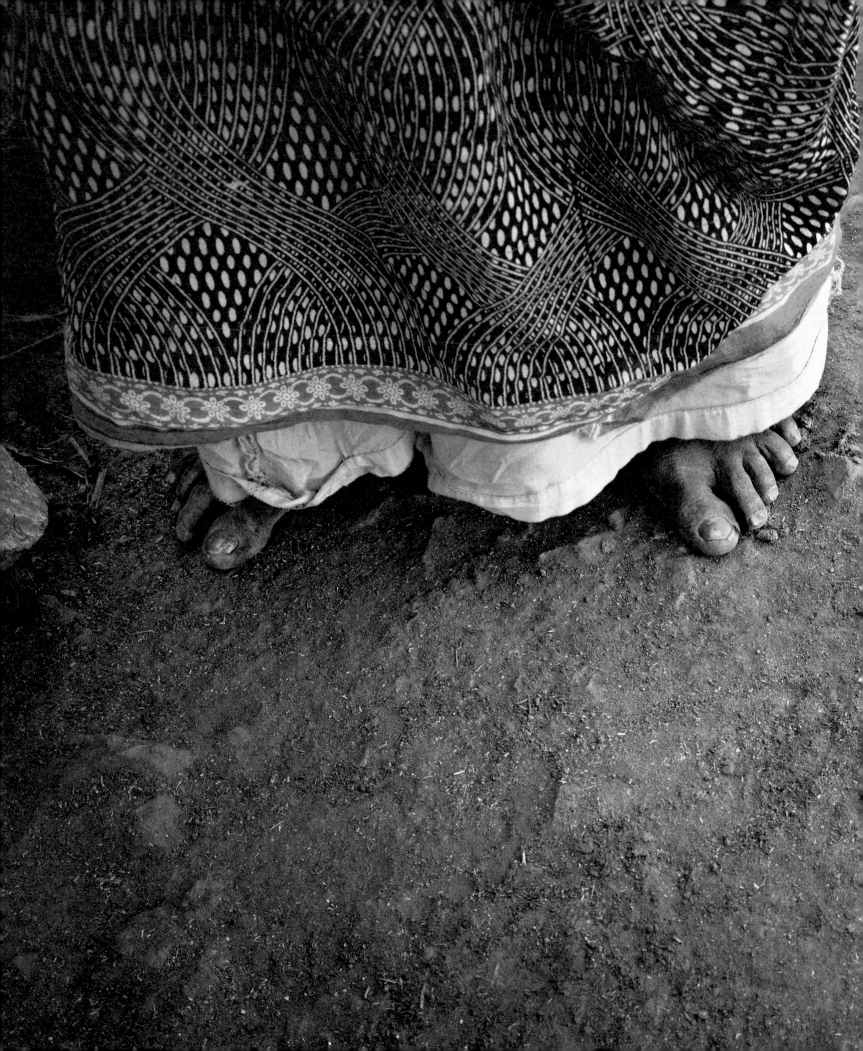

Narrative One

WOMEN, WOOD & BURNING

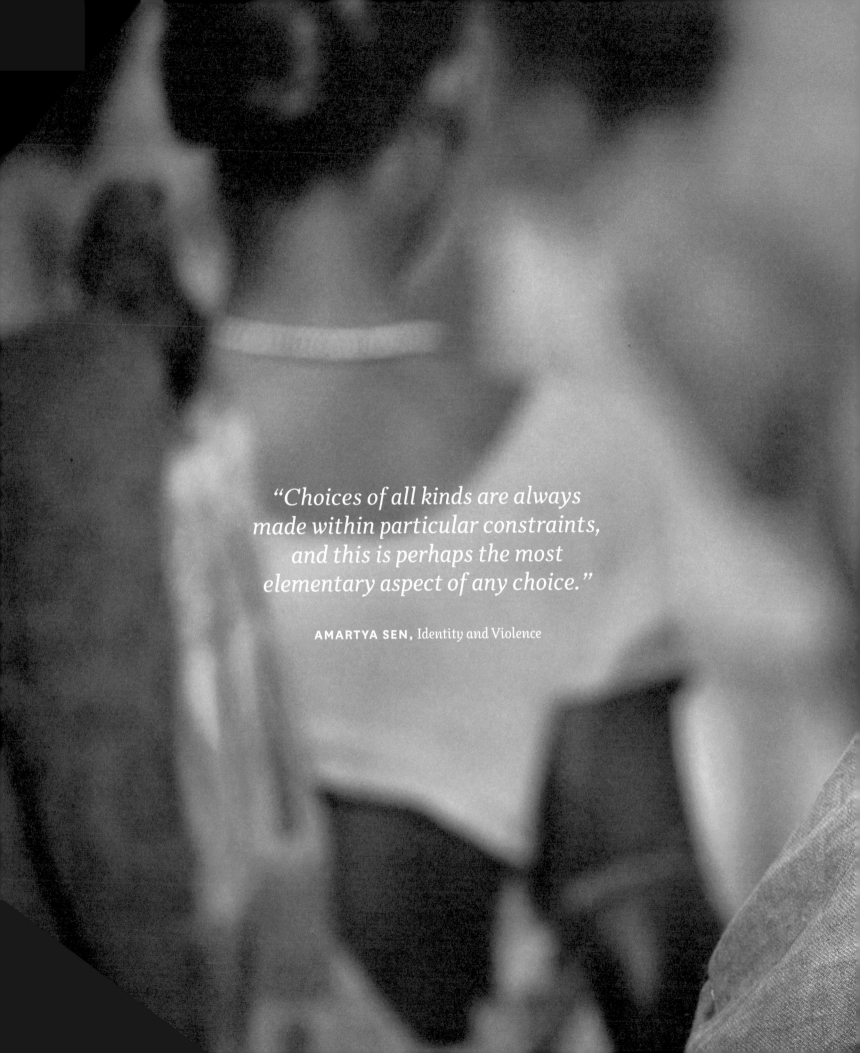

"Choices of all kinds are always made within particular constraints, and this is perhaps the most elementary aspect of any choice."

AMARTYA SEN, *Identity and Violence*

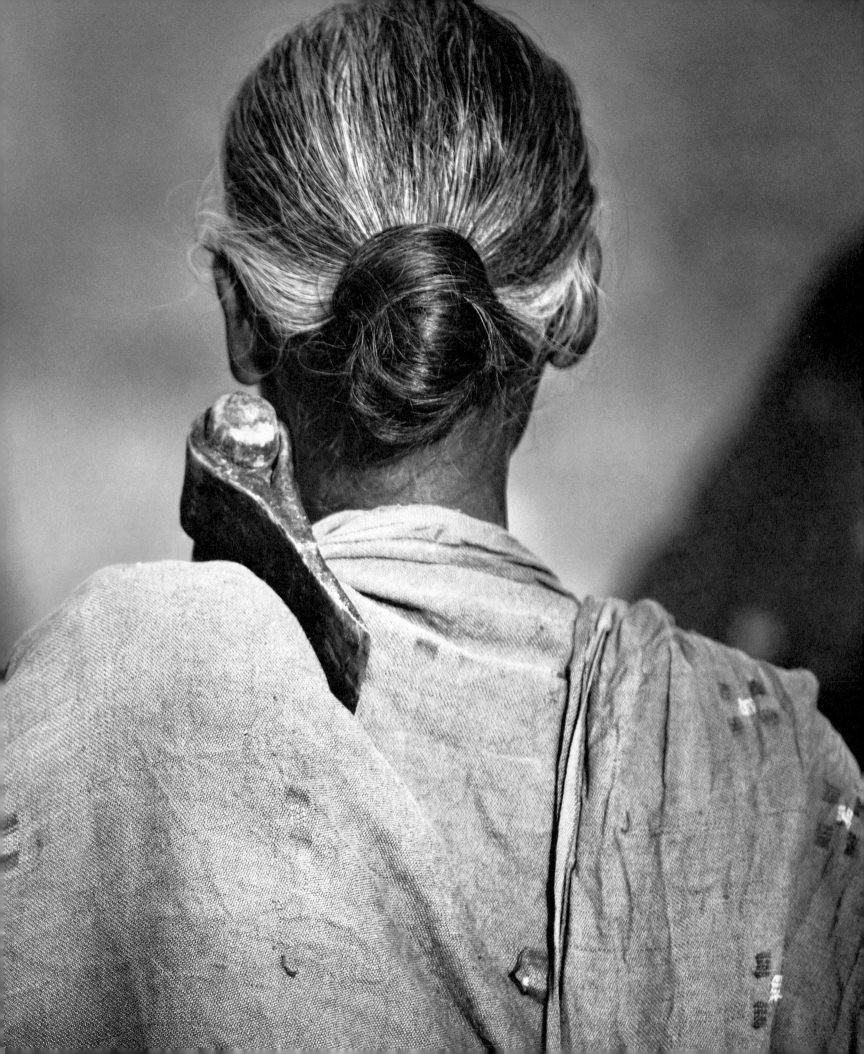

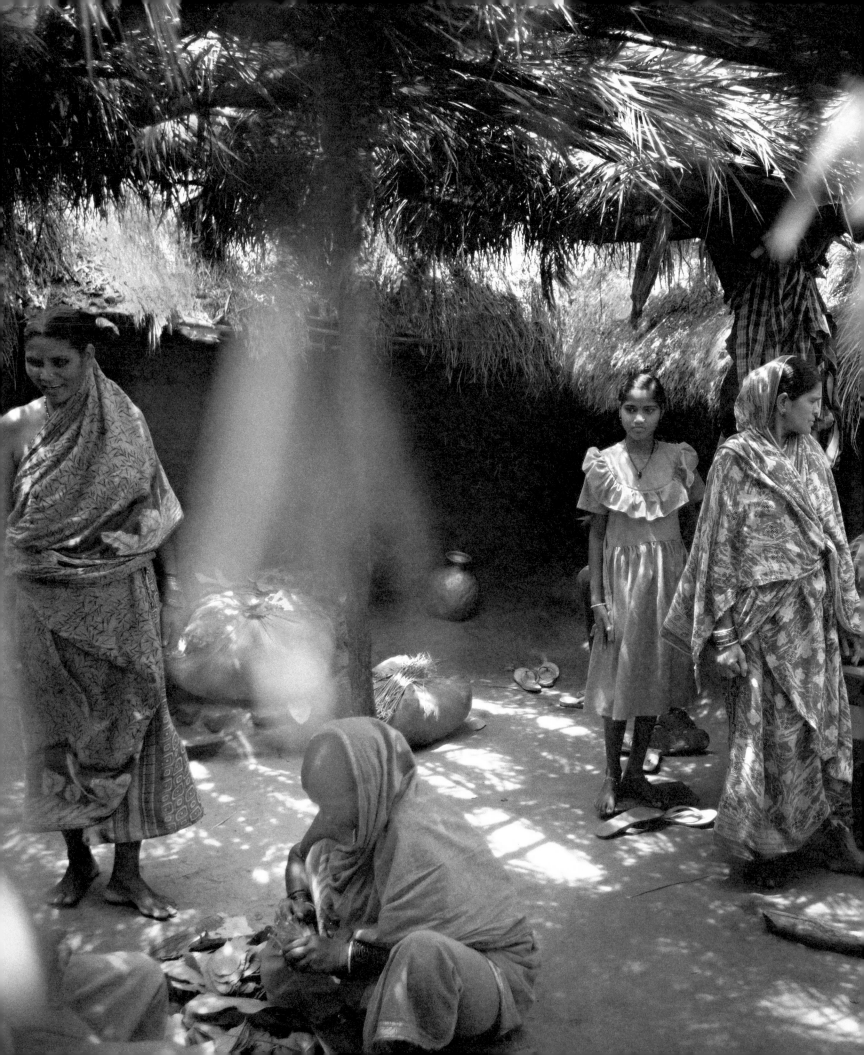

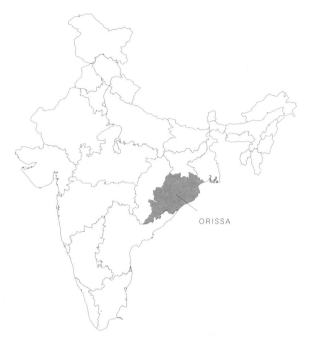

ORISSA

*Patchwork Lives in
the Satkosia Gorge*

COLLECTING WOOD FOR A FAMILY OF THIRTY

The Satkosia Gorge in the Angul district of Orissa
is home to tigers, elephants, and humans. Those who
live in the villages on the periphery of the Satkosia
forest routinely collect different types of forest
produce to supplement their incomes and to use
in their homes.

The family of potters that I met in 2012 in a village
close to the forest is no exception. The patriarch
of the family is in his 70s and his wife is a bit
younger. They have four grown sons, each with his
own family. The first son has eight children—three
daughters and five sons. The second son has three
daughters and two sons. The third son has only
two children—a son and a daughter. The fourth son
has three daughters and a son. When you include

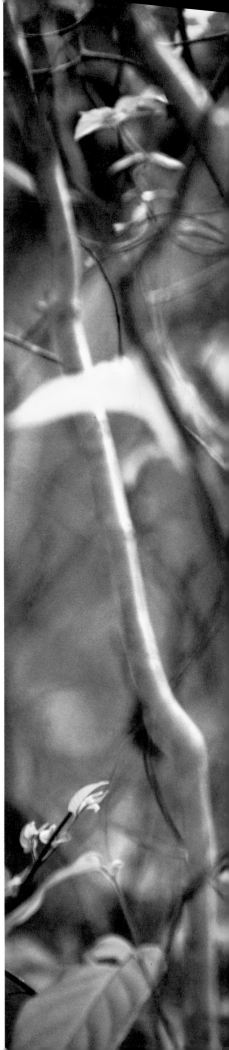

the wives of these four sons, the total comes to twenty-nine people. Then, when you add the most recent addition to the family—the twenty-year-old new bride of the oldest grandson—you have thirty members of this family living in the same house in four separate rooms circling a courtyard.

Collectively, they are engaged in a patchwork of daily wage labor (*majdoori*) during the agricultural season. They construct roads and buildings, collect Mahua flowers from the forest to make a local liquor, and prepare lands for government projects when those jobs are available. Occasionally, there is daily contractual work for the Forest Department.

During the non-agriculture season of April and May, women and children collect Tendu leaves from the forest. These leaves, used for rolling local cigarettes (*beedi*), are picked all day, and a bundle of 2,000 leaves earns workers 40 rupees (approximately $0.80 U.S. at the time of this writing). Two million people in Orissa collect Tendu leaves during these months, making it a significant source of income in the lean season, before the rains begin and agriculture work begins. So it is for our family of potters.

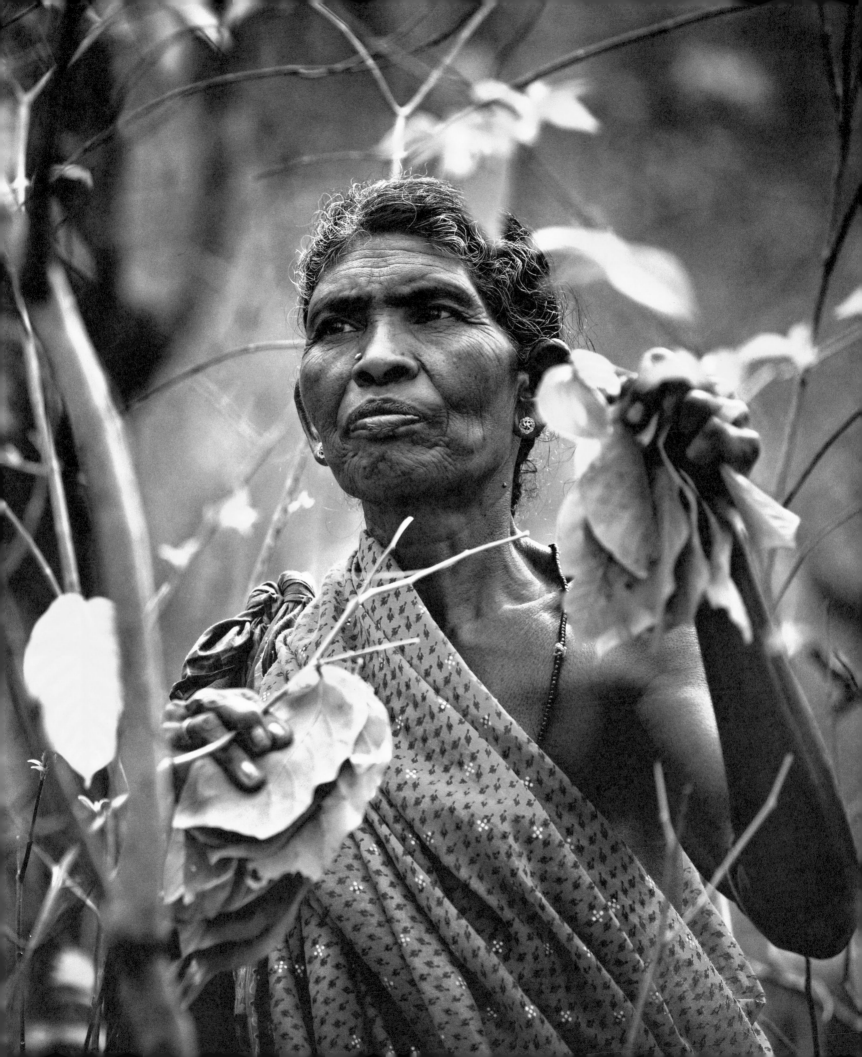

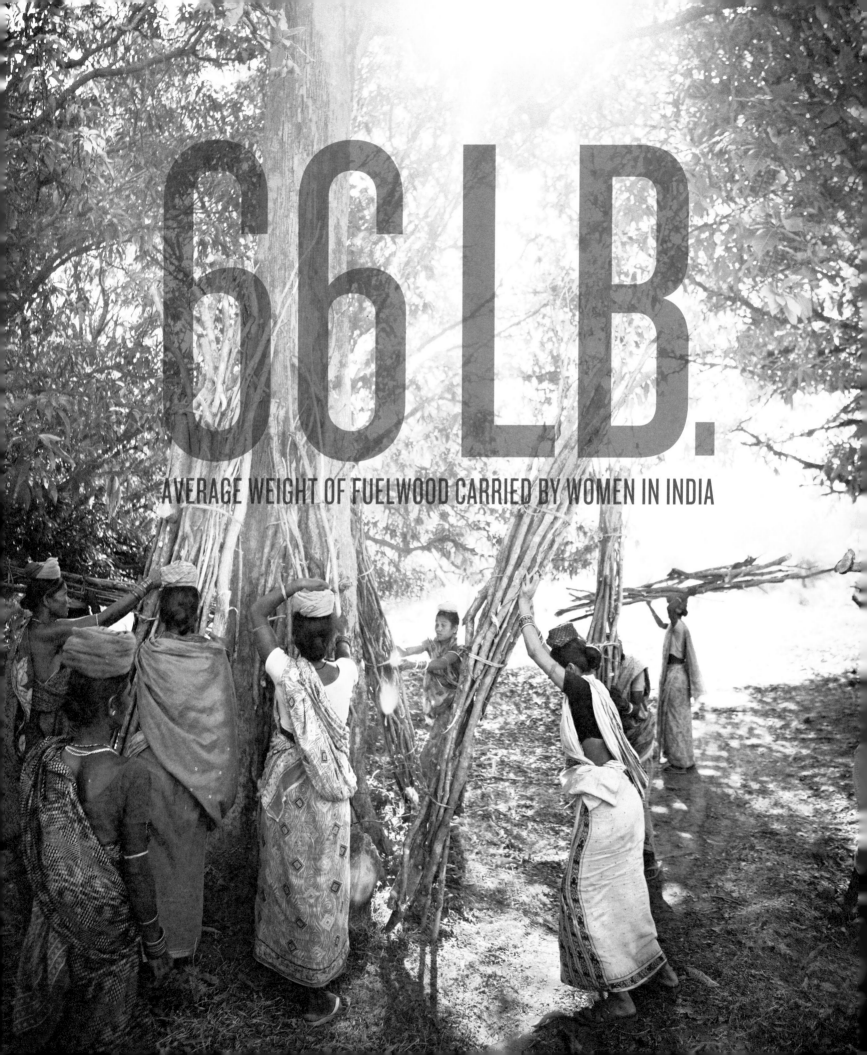

66 LB.

AVERAGE WEIGHT OF FUELWOOD CARRIED BY WOMEN IN INDIA

For thirty members of a family to make a living, you need this elaborate patchwork of jobs (one of the grandsons even owns a bicycle repair shop), forest-produce collection of all types, and much more. The patriarch of the house owns two acres of land on an upland slope near the forest. Uplands are not productive, however, and when divided among the four sons, it amounts to half an acre for each family. It is nearly impossible to feed a family from a tiny plot of unproductive upland farmland.

In contrast to what this family has, its needs are plenty. Women need twenty kilograms of wood daily to cook for their families—eighty kilograms every day for this collective family of thirty people. Once again, they go to the forest to bring this wood in every day. Just imagine bringing 176 pounds of wood a day from the forest, then burning it to cook, only to ingest smoke and particulate matter from incomplete combustion of wood.

This is the daily rhythm of this family, seven days a week. Each individual family has a wood-burning stove, some efficient and others not. In the realm of possibilities, the potter family is unable to afford or imagine owning anything other than a wood-burning stove. When you have thirty people to feed daily on a patchwork of livelihoods that are all at the margins of a local economy, it is prudent to rely on a nearby forest and women who are compliant to bring large amounts of wood on their backs to cook and feed. Women in this family were not an exception. They invited me to walk with them to the forest on their next collection. I agreed without hesitation. By 6 a.m. the next morning, photographer Mark Katzman and I were ready in the village to join them.

A MORNING FOR COLLECTING

The wives of the four brothers met us, and we began walking through the village toward the forest as they called out to other women to join in wood collection. Soon we were walking behind a group of eleven women and a dog heading toward the forest about three kilometers away. Trailing at the end was a woman with a twisted right foot, limping. We were heading to a patch of forest designated for this village, and managed and regulated by its community. A woman in a pink saree with an axe over her shoulder walked in a single line with others in blue, bright yellowish green with patterns, and purple. The last woman, with her right leg bent, struggled to keep up with the rest. The sun was already hot and rising.

As we approached the forest opening, a woman kneeled down in a quick bow to the trees ahead. I was not expecting this sudden reverence and respect, displayed as it was just prior to the aggressive chopping that was soon to follow. Perhaps it was partly a gesture of gratitude for the abundant wood in such close proximity to their village, but also partly an apology for the imminent reckless extraction of their forest, this temple of wood.

The women soon put their various materials, including a few water bottles, in one place, then spread themselves outward in a circular fashion into the forest. As they fanned out, they began hunting for wood that they liked, some fallen and dried and ready to gather. Other wood was in large fallen branches that had to be axed.

They walked quickly and with purpose around the forest, breaking sticks and chopping fallen trees, still talking to each other from afar, shouting across the thicket. Ringing in the air all around their voices was a high-pitched sound of crickets, along with the steady cracking sound of wood. Morning parakeets flew from one tree to another. Relentlessly chopping, the women kept up the pace, without resting, for nearly an hour. They had other chores waiting to be finished in the village.

We watched them split wood on all sides. When the women were satisfied with the size of the splintered wood, they dragged the pieces to a central place, assembling the wood in bundles. Even as gathering was going on, some women started preparing ropes using the thin bark of a thick creeper to tie the wood bundles. They tied them on both ends with tight knots, twisting the fresh ropes. Their daily exercise was evident in their sinewy, torquing arms.

When the bundles were ready for transport, those tasked with carrying the most weight—easily 100-pound bundles—received help from the others, who lifted and placed them on twisted cloths sitting on their heads like nests.

In watching them, it was clear that this was a lot of weight, a significant burden that surely strained their necks, backs, and legs. It is difficult to rationalize that women preferred to do this daily. What other options did the women in the potter family have, with thirty members to cook for every day? What is their exit?

THE BODY BENEATH [1-5]

Women have been observed carrying up to 70 kg. (154 lb.) of fuelwood over long distances. The health impacts of "head-bearing" or "head-loading" fuelwood are significant, particularly for children. It has been shown to lead to arthritis in the spine, especially the neck, as well as long-term neck and back pain. Head-loading also causes abnormal wear on the body's cartilage and bones, leading to degenerative joint disease. Greatly under-recognized is the risk of uterine prolapse from carrying heavy loads of fuelwood, water, and fodder, as women are culture-bound to do soon after childbirth.

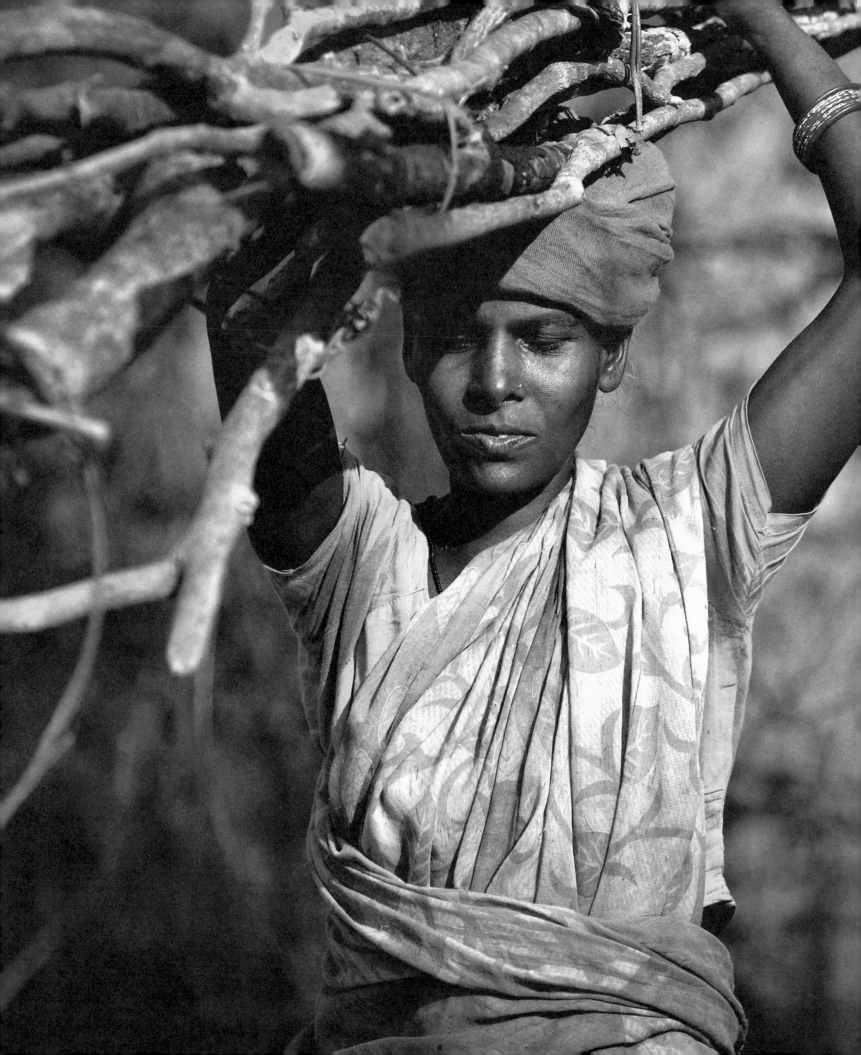

"ADAPTIVE PREFERENCES ARE FORMED WITHOUT ONE'S CONTROL OR AWARENESS, BY A CAUSAL MECHANISM THAT ISN'T OF ONE'S OWN CHOOSING."

MARTHA C. NUSSBAUM, *Women and Human Development*

The women were now ready, lined up with freshly cut wood hoisted and perched on the soft cloths on their heads. They began walking out of the forest toward the village. With all that weight and the heat, they had to stop at least once before arriving in their village. The woman with the limp took her time, falling behind the others. Eventually, they stopped under a large Mahua tree, rested, drank water, and talked about the morning. In the midst of that drudgery, there was laughter and banter. All their bundles, those tall structures, rested vertically in a circle around the giant trunk of a Mahua tree. After fifteen minutes of rest, they were ready to return to the village. When they did, the women peeled off as they approached their homes, just as they had when going into the forest. Three to four hours later, we were back at the potters' home with fresh bundles of wood that would dry for several more days before being used.

FIRES TO LIGHT

It was now around 11 a.m., time for lunch to be prepared. The women began assembling wood in the stoves. The new bride, several months pregnant, was already cooking in a small kitchen on a traditional mud stove. The older women cooked in the open in the courtyard, with some of the other men assembled in the periphery. Some were counting and bundling Tendu leaves along with younger girls of the household. This was Tendu season, and there was daily collection of bundles. (Had it not been Tendu season, these girls would be collecting wood or hay, or doing some other chore.)

The toughest task was being done by the new bride—cooking in a closed space, which she did for two hours. Her young husband proudly proclaimed that she does that for two hours in the morning and in the evening. In her pregnant state, she was inhaling all that heat and smoke for four hours a day. The older women still gathered wood, but at least they cooked outside. They did not have to suffer the close confines of an indoor kitchen combined with a traditional stove. It seemed almost as if they'd put in their time, and did not need to suffer as much as this young bride. No one seemed to bother about the baby, who will surely suffer from all the particulate matter this young woman was inhaling.

The women in this extended family household held very unequal positions, as evidenced in seeing the young bride in sweltering heat enveloped in smoke in that kitchen. Then there were children, readying bundles, preparing for a life of carrying wood and cooking with wood.

What choices do these women have but to support a family of thirty people whose livelihoods are like a fragile quilt, constantly being repaired and tenuously held together? How does one intervene to address the energy choices in this delicately balanced household? What incentives could we provide for these women not to go to the forest and meet their household energy needs in a gender-unequal decision space? This is the challenge of stove programs and clean-energy interventions that aspire to bring energy security to the poor. ✤

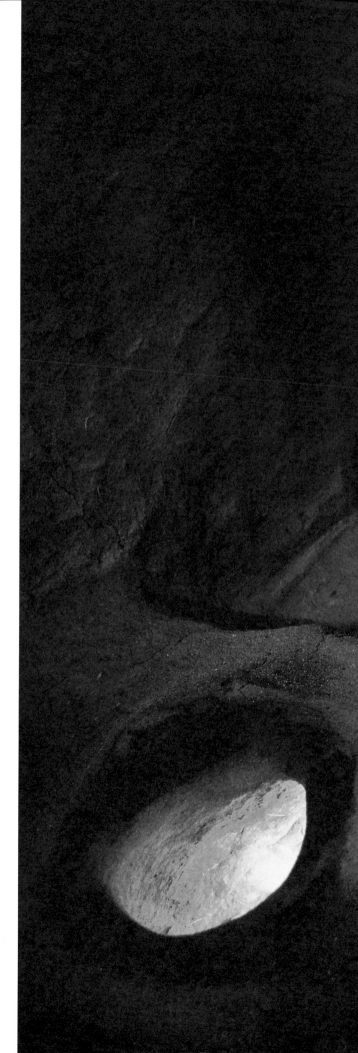

VULNERABLE AT BIRTH [6-9]

73 GRAMS

The amount by which babies born to mothers using high-polluting fuels are lighter than babies born to mothers using low-polluting fuels

50%

Amount of the 1.24 million annual child deaths under the age of 5 that are caused by pneumonia from inhaling particulate matter from indoor air pollution

20%

How much more likely babies exposed to first-trimester carbon dioxide are to experience intrauterine growth retardation

872,000

Number of children under the age of 5 who suffer from acute lower respiratory infections related to household air pollution

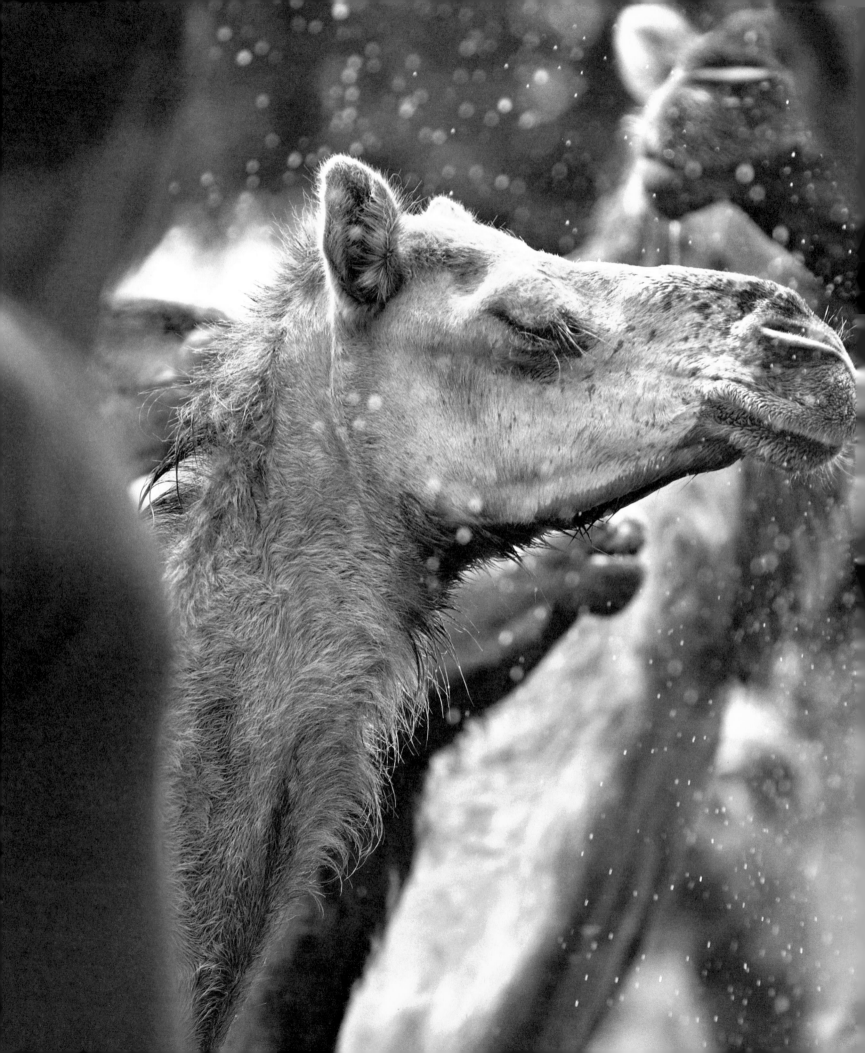

Narrative Two

LAND & LIVING

Making ends meet with only buffalo
has become difficult.
Enter demand for charcoal.

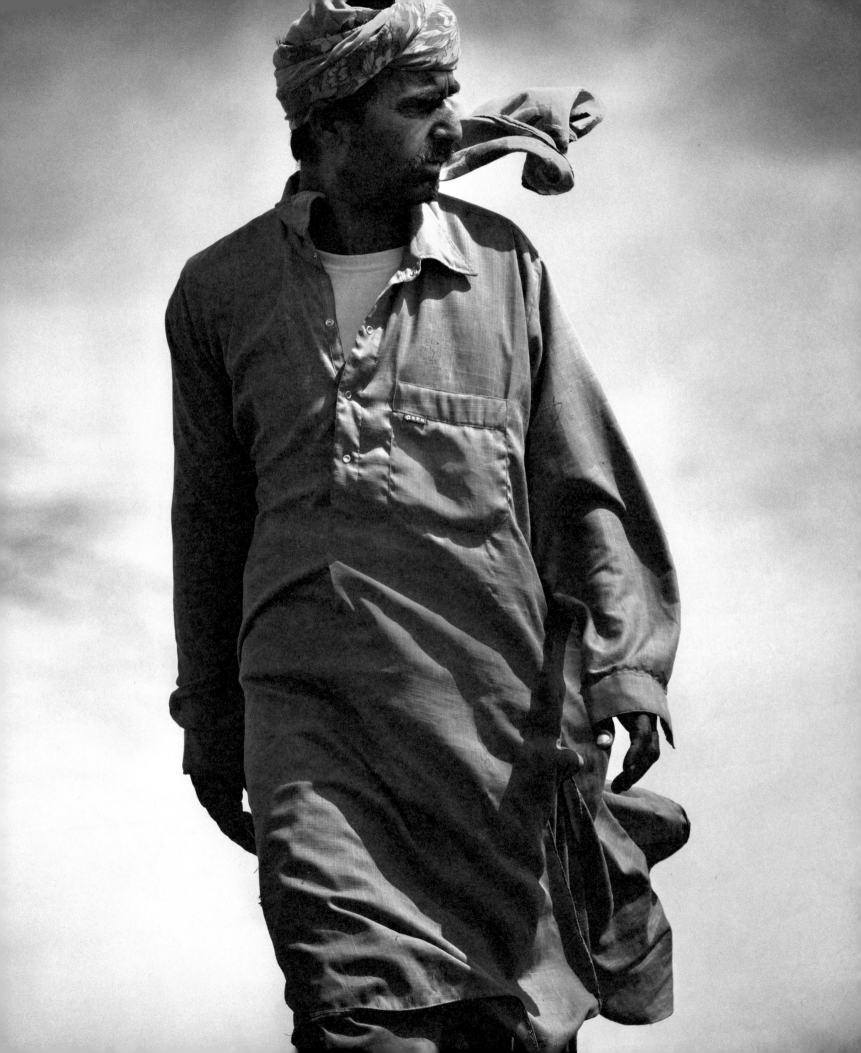

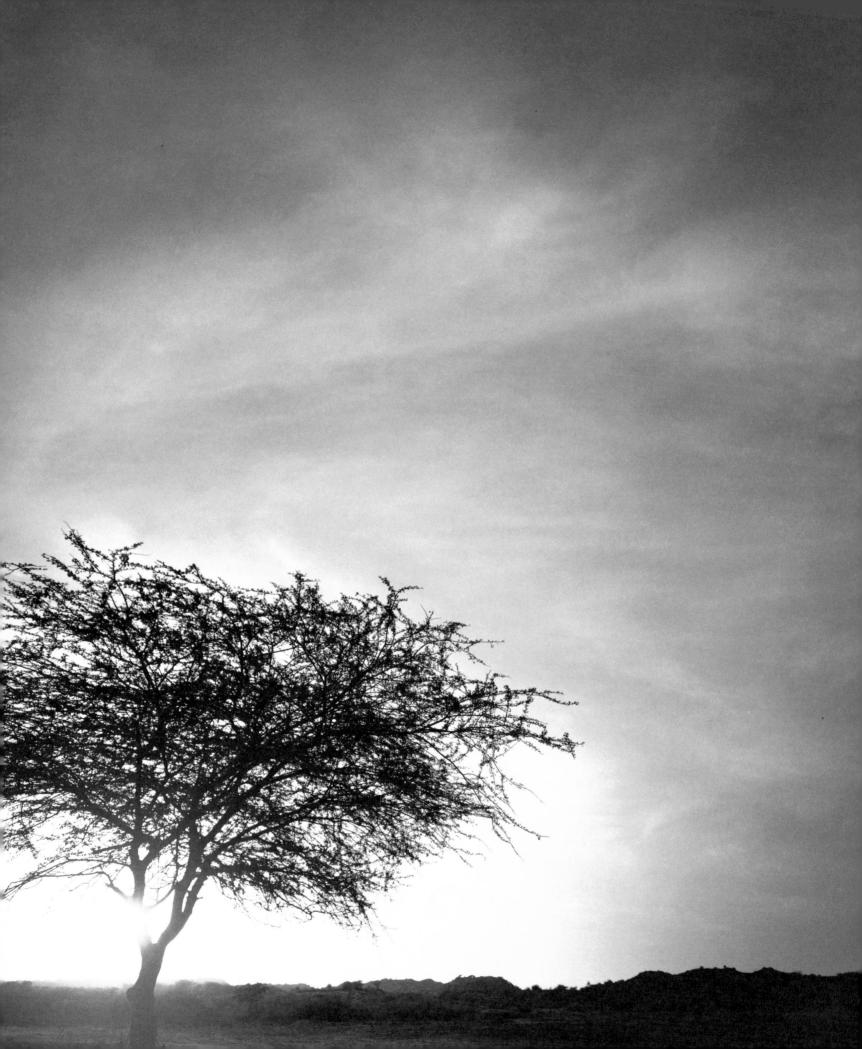

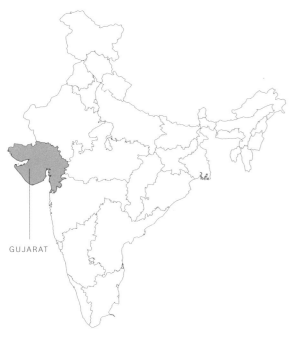

NARRATIVE TWO

The Paradox of Kutch

ABUNDANT WOOD, FRAYED LIVELIHOODS

Kutch, located in the state of Gujarat, is the
largest district in all of India—and ground zero
for understanding the dynamic complexity of energy
poverty, people, environment, local ecosystems,
and fragile livelihoods. A granular, telling picture
of energy, poverty, and the environment emerges
by exploring two stories within the pastoral villages
of Abdasha Taluka of Kutch and the Banni grasslands.
In very different ways, we see how two communities
respond to the invasive species *Prosopis juliflora,*
a woody plant seen in the photograph at left. In
the first case, its massive emergence threatens a
traditional livelihood. In the second, it provides
a new one. But at a cost.

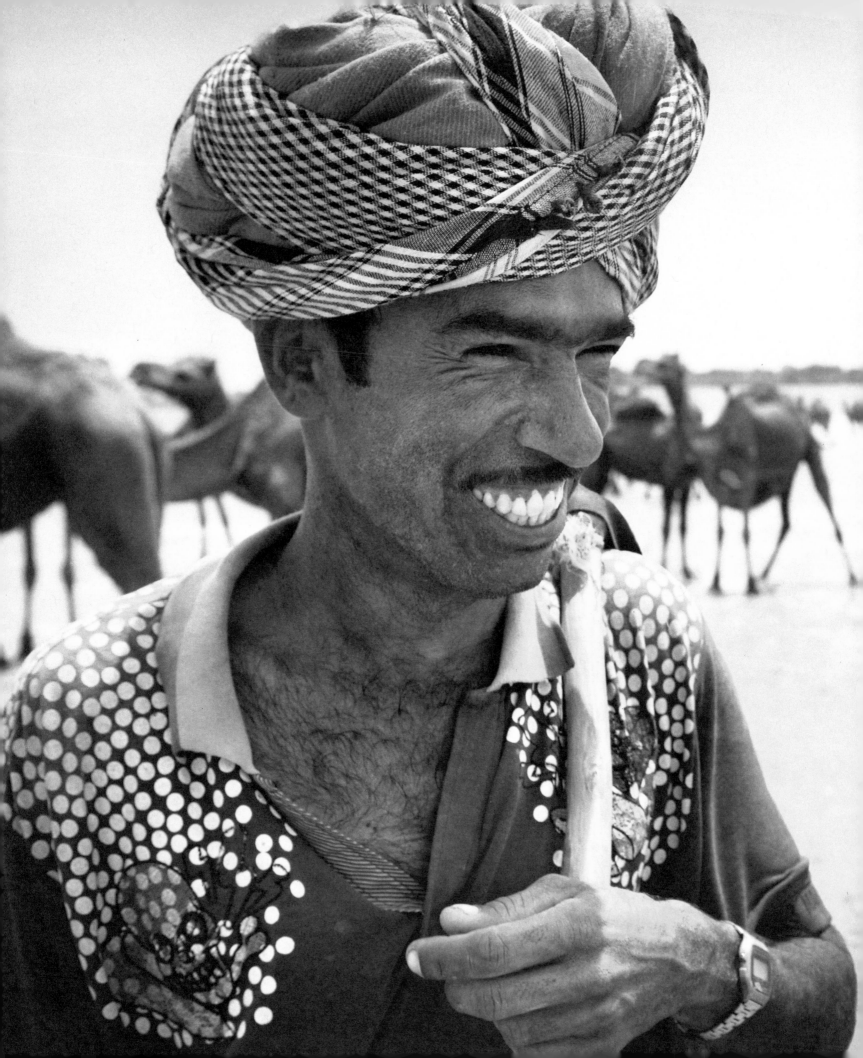

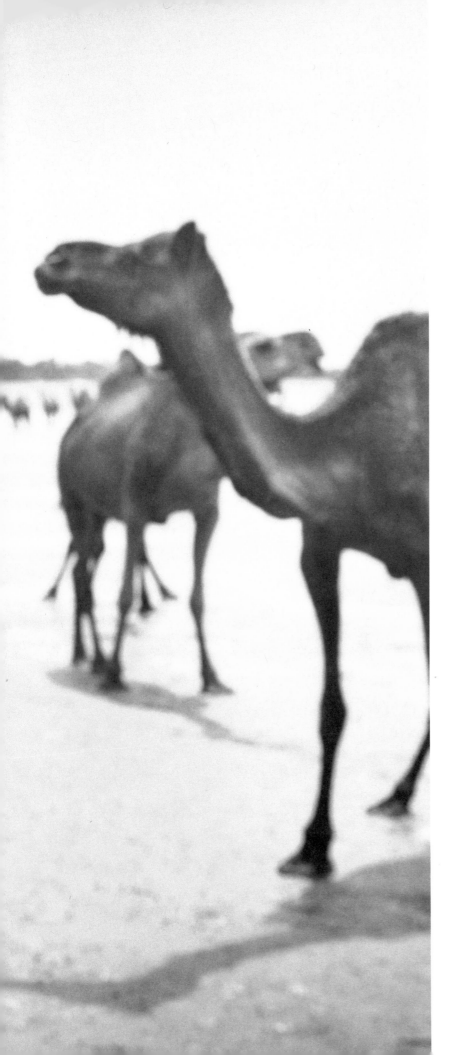

FAKIRANI JAT CAMEL HERDERS, MANGROVES, AND FUEL

For the past twenty years, the nongovernmental organization Sahjeevan has been working to organize the Maldharis, the seminomadic pastoralists with buffalos, cows, and camels, to regain control of the basic inputs required for sustainable and stable livelihoods. These inputs are from grasslands or mangroves, depending on the region of Kutch.

Through Sahjeevan, Mark Katzman and I met two distinct groups of Jat Muslim herders—those who own buffalo and cow and live in the Banni grasslands, and those who own and breed Kharai camels. The lives of the latter group, Fakirani Jats, are delicately perched between the mangrove forests on the coast and the terrestrial ecosystems of Kutch. In an oft-repeated pattern, these men drive their camels through the intertidal areas into the mangroves so that the animals may feed, graze, and breed; the men return back to their villages every three days to seek fresh water for their camels.

On a trip during April 2012, we arrived at the edge of the estuary and waited for three herders to emerge from a distant mangrove forest. The water was high, and the mangroves in the distance were submerged, with only their tops peeking out. After an hour, the tide receded, and a faint train of camels began extending out of the mangroves. Another hour later, we heard grunting and calling, as two men cajoled and coaxed neck-deep camels through the estuary and onto land.

These camels and men were returning after several days in the mangroves, a rich source of fodder and food supporting a lifestyle of camel breeding and selling. Fakirani Jat families care for their own camels, but also earn income by taking care of camels loaned to them by other herding families. Out of the 100 camels we saw on this trip, thirty were on loan to these Maldharis—earning the men an additional 1,200 rupees. In Kutch, camels are bred and sold every two or three years for approximately 6,000 rupees for a 3-year-old camel.

The mangroves in these estuaries of the Arabian Sea provide a fragile living for the Jats between sea and land. They do not farm—camel herding is their sole living. With such a variable income, the availability of mangroves is critical.

Their villages and homes are simple, stripped-down huts made of reed and grass atop rolling mounds of sand. The sole exception to this ordinary scene is the beautiful and ornate embroidery and jewelry adorning the village's women, who remain in the village while the men herd. Their beautifully sewn clothes and ornaments are in direct contrast to their simple homes and harsh existence.

87

MANGROVE FORESTS IN THE TROPICS HAVE DECLINED SIGNIFICANTLY, BY

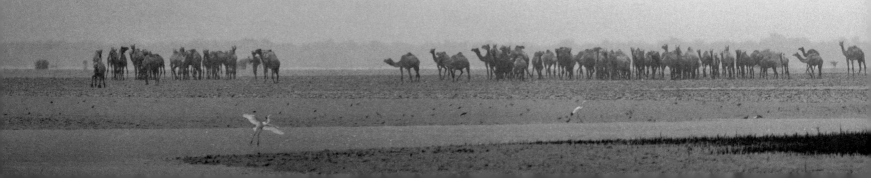

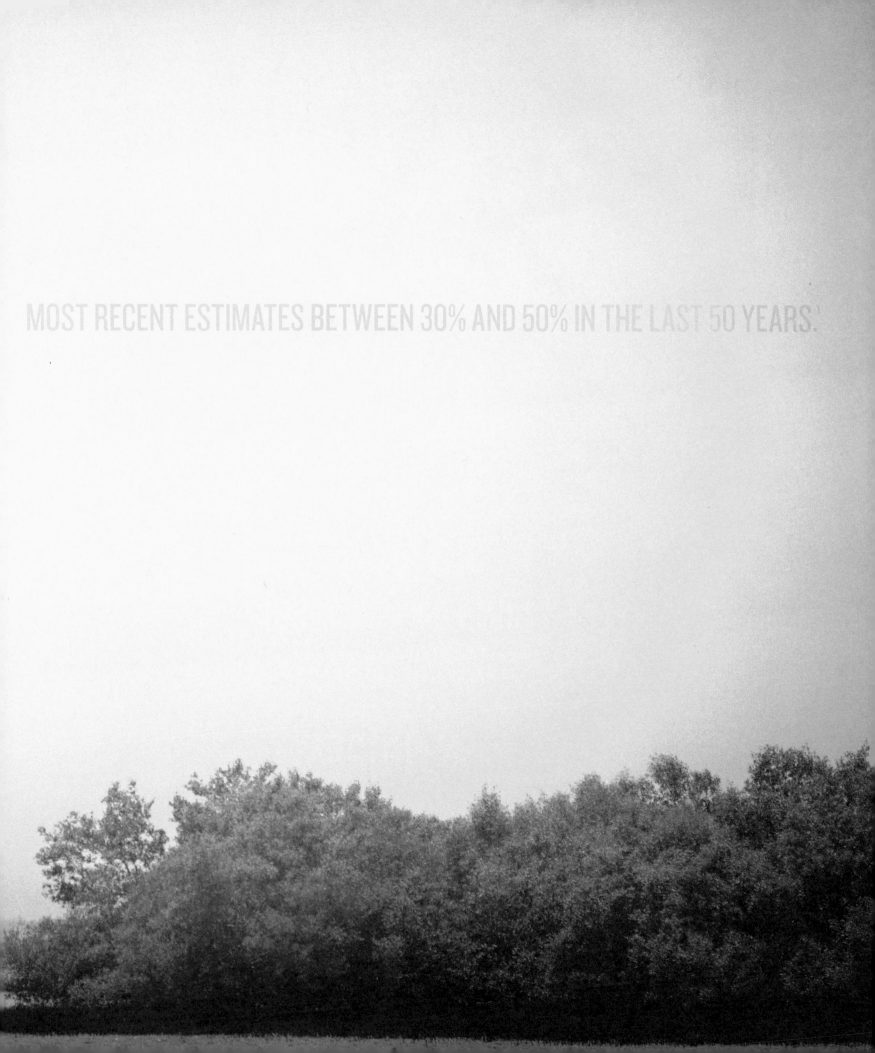

MOST RECENT ESTIMATES BETWEEN 30% AND 50% IN THE LAST 50 YEARS.

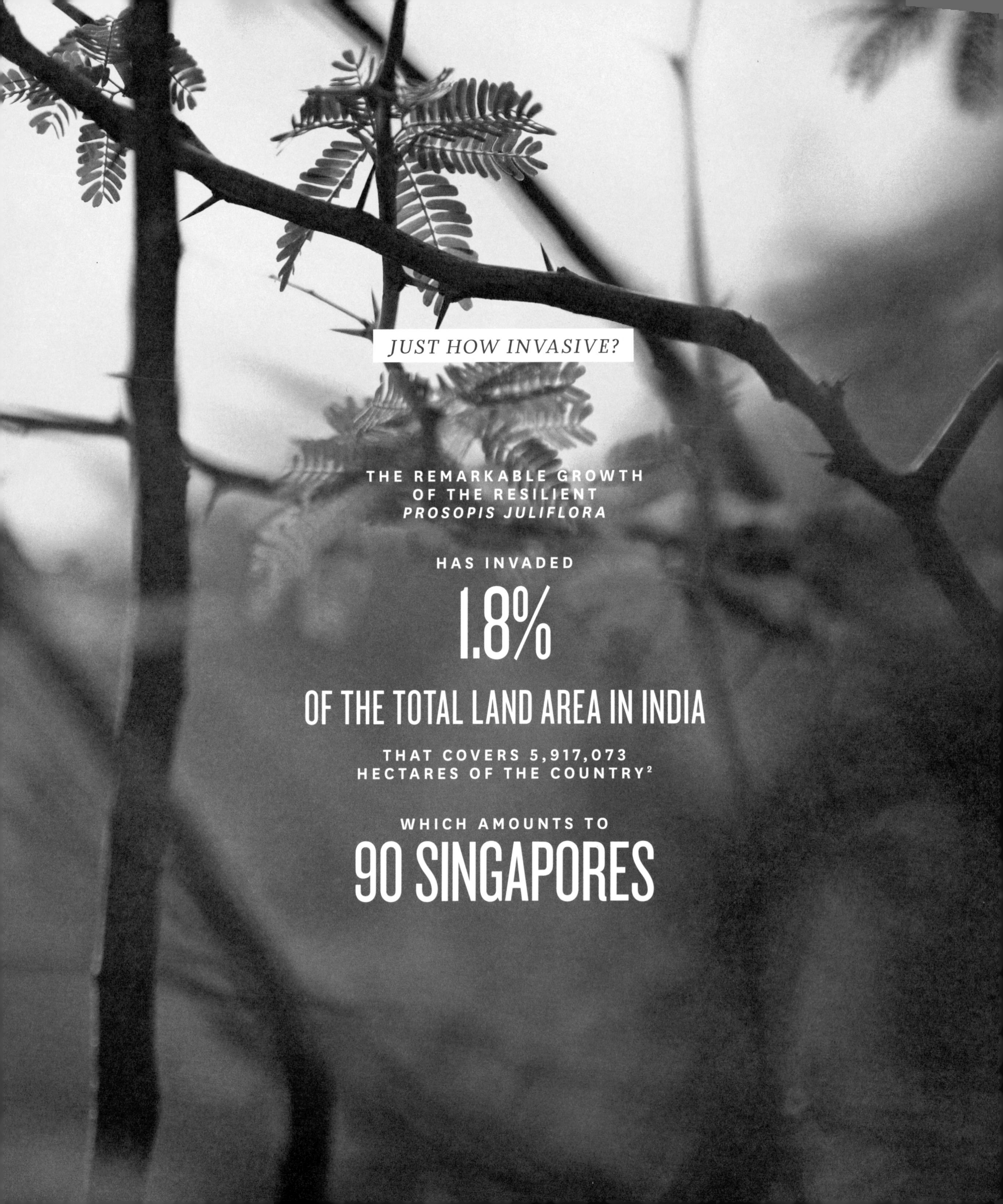

THE REMARKABLE GROWTH
OF THE RESILIENT
PROSOPIS JULIFLORA

HAS INVADED

1.8%

OF THE TOTAL LAND AREA IN INDIA

THAT COVERS 5,917,073
HECTARES OF THE COUNTRY[2]

WHICH AMOUNTS TO

90 SINGAPORES

Kharai camel herding is under considerable pressure from declining mangrove forests and other grazing areas on land. Mangrove forests in the tropics have declined significantly, by most recent estimates between 30% and 50% in the last fifty years.[3] A decline in mangrove forests is not only a shock to the livelihoods of Jat camel herders, but because they are carbon-dense forests, their decline generates carbon emissions, affecting other ecosystem services.

On land, the Jats are also experiencing declines in grasses good for camel grazing, because aggressive growth of the invasive woody plant *Prosopis juliflora* is crowding them out. Paradoxically, this troublesome species—known locally as *Gando bawal*, or "mad tree"—makes for an excellent fuel for household cooking and heating. It is abundant and easy to light, and is often used by the women inside these simple homes.

Certainly, the challenge to provide clean-energy systems is further compounded in Kutch, when we connect fragile camel herding livelihoods, disappearing mangroves, and fast-spreading, abundant, and mad *Prosopis juliflora*. What incentives remain for a Fakirani Jat family to replace this aggressive wood with a cleaner fuel? What incentives remain for families to shift to an efficient stove when fuel is so abundant? *Gando bawal* is spreading in the Banni grasslands of Kutch, changing the livelihoods of other pastoral communities as well. Its invasion has reduced the potential for grazing grass cover from 1,610 square kilometers to a mere 350 square kilometers.[4] The irony in this invasion is evident in a different Jat community that herds milk-producing buffalo in the Banni grasslands.

CASE 2: JAT NOMADIC BUFFALO HERDERS
Deep inside the Banni grasslands, Jat families—women and children included—produce charcoal. This charcoal ends up in urban and peri-urban households and small commercial restaurants throughout India. These Maldharis are primarily buffalo-rearing and traditionally rely on the grasslands to produce milk. Income from charcoal is supplementary, but robust. These Jat families capitalize on the synergies between demand for charcoal in urban India, and ecosystem transformations in Banni grasslands suitable for charcoal making.

These grasslands have declined in quality and productivity from a combination of factors: a steady erosion of traditional grazing rights that Banni residents claim they had for more than 200 years, along with state intervention to stem land degradation through the introduction of *Prosopis juliflora*, which, according to the people there, is now choking the grasslands. Many indigenous grasses critical for buffalo and cattle grazing and milk production have been declining. Making ends meet with only buffalo has become difficult. Enter demand for charcoal from the outside, and the high-quality charcoal potential from the invasive *Gando bawal*.

The possibility to turn this invasive plant pest into shiny charcoal for additional income was not lost on this Jat family on that April afternoon in 2012, as we walked into their village. They had deployed everyone in the family to make charcoal, with the head of the family supervising.

Charcoal making is a pyrolytic process where wood is heated until it carbonizes. It is strenuous, time-consuming, and dangerous. Pyrolysis happens slowly, without oxygen, and produces not only charcoal, but also harmful gases—including carbon monoxide, carbon dioxide, methane, and ethane.

In scanning the scene in that Jat village, it was evident that making charcoal to meet the energy demands of a distant household was taking its toll on the health of women and children engaged in the production. Smoke was rising from brownish black ground and covering perhaps ten large piles of invasive mesquite wood spread all around in this large open yard just outside the village settlement. In their midst were women covered from head to toe, veiled, ghostly, and shielding themselves from this continuous smoke. Children were lingering near their mothers, mostly not bothered by the smoke, except when the blowing wind would direct the smoke right into their faces. Women were busy, focused, and tending to these piles of burning wood that were covered in a thick layer of mud, with straw sandwiched between the mud and wood. They were ensuring a slow pyrolysis and good charcoal. Some of the women stoked the fires beneath the mound, and regulated the heat by closing and opening vents on the side of these piles. These piles had been lit the day before, and they'd been slowly burning all night. Other women prepared new piles of wood to be covered in straw and mud and lit. Others chopped the wood into the right size. Men watched over the

ANOTHER INVADER [5-7]

Like *Prosopis*, a plant known as *Lantana camara* has been purposefully or accidentally introduced to native forests—and it's spreading rapidly. It currently occupies more than 5 million hectares in Australia, 13 million in India, and 2 million in South Africa. The species has many features that allow it to successfully spread and dominate native habitats and dramatically transform ecosystems: it aggressively sequesters soil nutrients and water and outcompetes most native plant species; it releases toxic chemicals into the soil that hinder the growth of other plants in its vicinity; and it produces abundant seeds that can travel long distances when consumed by birds. The plant has long-term negative effects on forest ecosystems—threatening biodiversity, agriculture, livestock, and human health—but because some of the *Lantana* species is useful for fuelwood in the short term, there is little motivation to manage its growth.
—*Tiffany Knight, Associate Professor, Department of Biology, Washington University in St. Louis*

EVERY YEAR

500,000

PEOPLE ON THE PLANET DIE

FROM THE EFFECTS OF OUTDOOR AIR POLLUTION PRODUCED FROM COOKING WITH SOLID FUELS.[8]

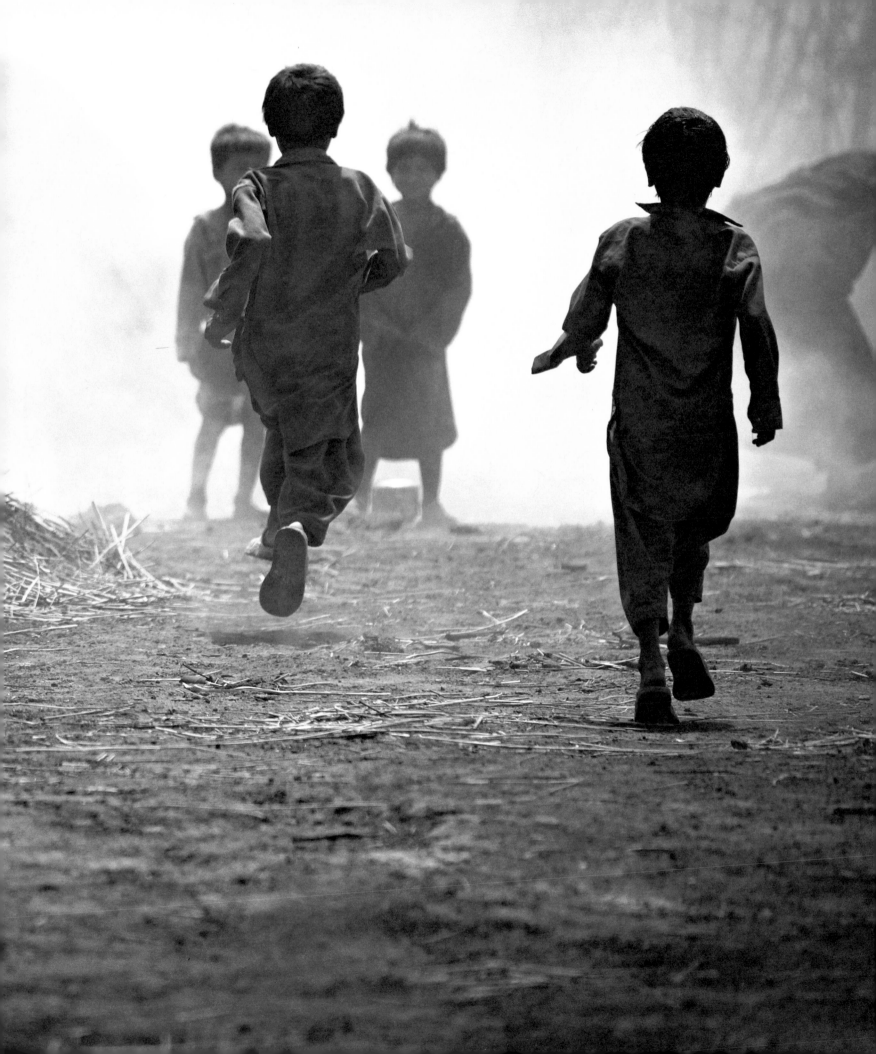

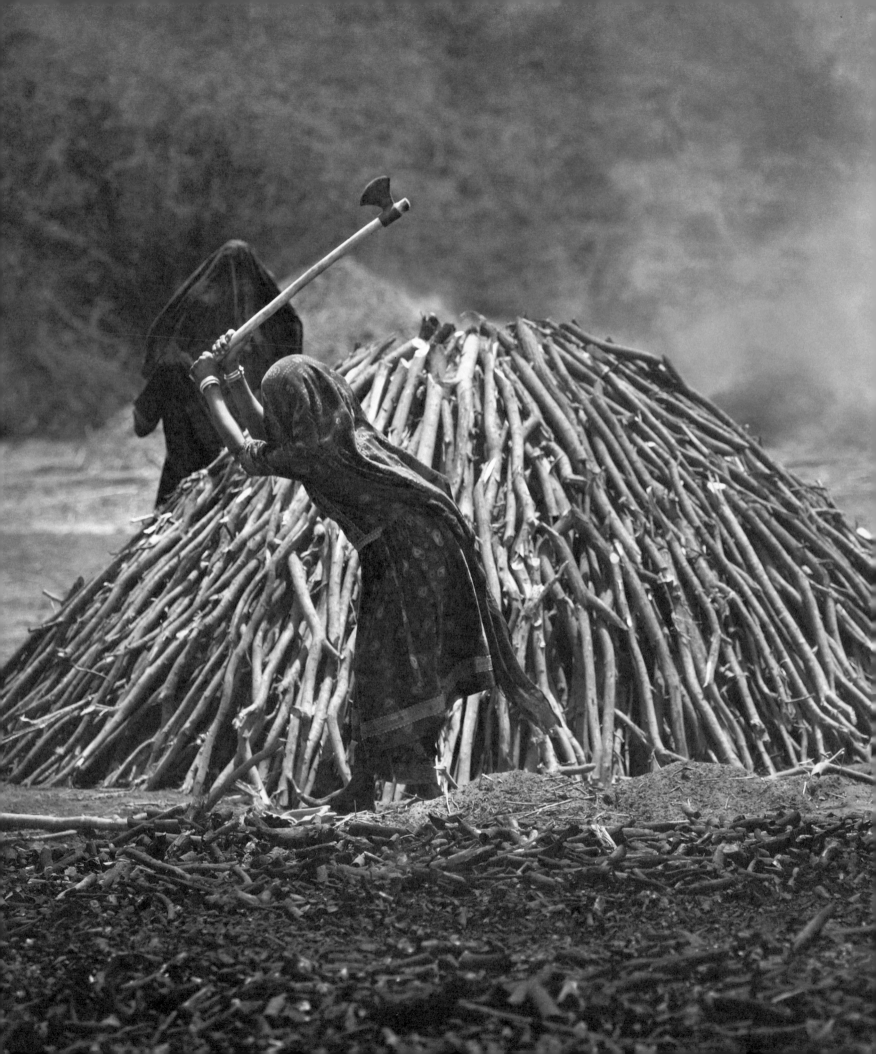

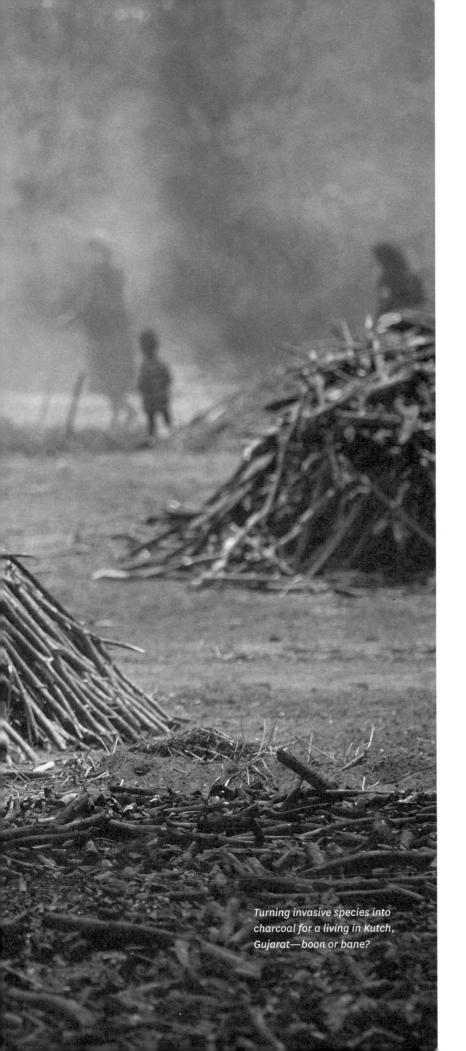

Turning invasive species into charcoal for a living in Kutch, Gujarat—boon or bane?

burning and smoking piles. Smoke swirled as the wind blew and covered everyone in its path. In the background were green *Gando bawal* trees standing as a reminder of the raw source of this charcoal.

It will take five days for this Jat family to produce eleven to twelve bags weighing forty kilograms apiece from each of the burning piles. Each bag will be sold for 200 rupees by this family, and will surely increase in price as the charcoal moves to markets. Working eight-hour days, if not more, the women will soon start assembling new piles of wood. As long as *Prosopis* is there, and demand for charcoal is there, life goes on deep in the Banni grasslands for these Jat women toiling in the heat of summer. If milk from the Banni buffalo is not abundant, there is the demand for shiny black charcoal from bustling markets supplying to homes where it will be burned once again, affecting the lives of different women and children. The only cost is women's labor, and their health. The wood is free, invasive, and abundant.

Charcoal production could soon be seen as supplementing income from milk production, perhaps making it the primary occupation if livelihoods from milk production become untenable. This could well be the case if people depend on the invasive plant species and are reluctant to control it for the additional income it provides through charcoal. Charcoal making could both transform the local ecology and completely shift the traditional livelihoods of the Banni people. And given the emissions from production, it is certain to adversely impact women, children, and the environment. All of this was evident in the dark and eerie scene I witnessed in this Jat village.

Our challenge is to intervene in this causal chain of declining productivity of land in Kutch, of increasing dependence on alternative livelihoods such as supplying the charcoal to energy-impoverished urban masses. To address the health of people and the climate from solid fuel burning—first in the making of it, and second at the household level as it's burned—we need sustainable livelihoods and productive agricultural systems, in addition to better combustion and improved stoves. We also need alternative sources of energy that are viable for the urban masses and the rural poor.

The poor of Banni, however, have abundant fuelwood that they are able to use in their homes, as I observed in their kitchens. But they are exporting it in the form of charcoal to the rest of India. How do we convince them to move to cleaner fuels and efficient combustion? This is our singular challenge: to understand the feedback mechanisms in a complex system of social, economic, ecological, and cultural processes. ❖

95

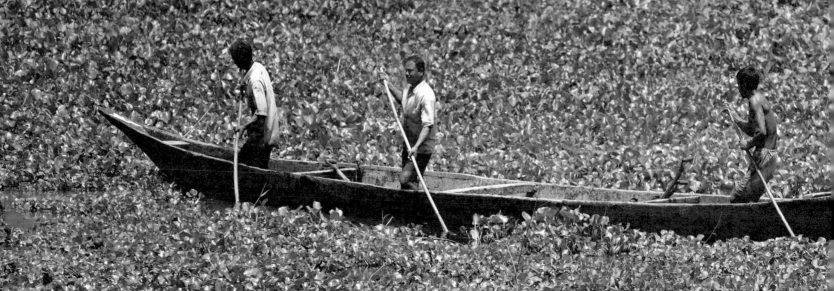

Narrative Three

STALLED BY TRADITION

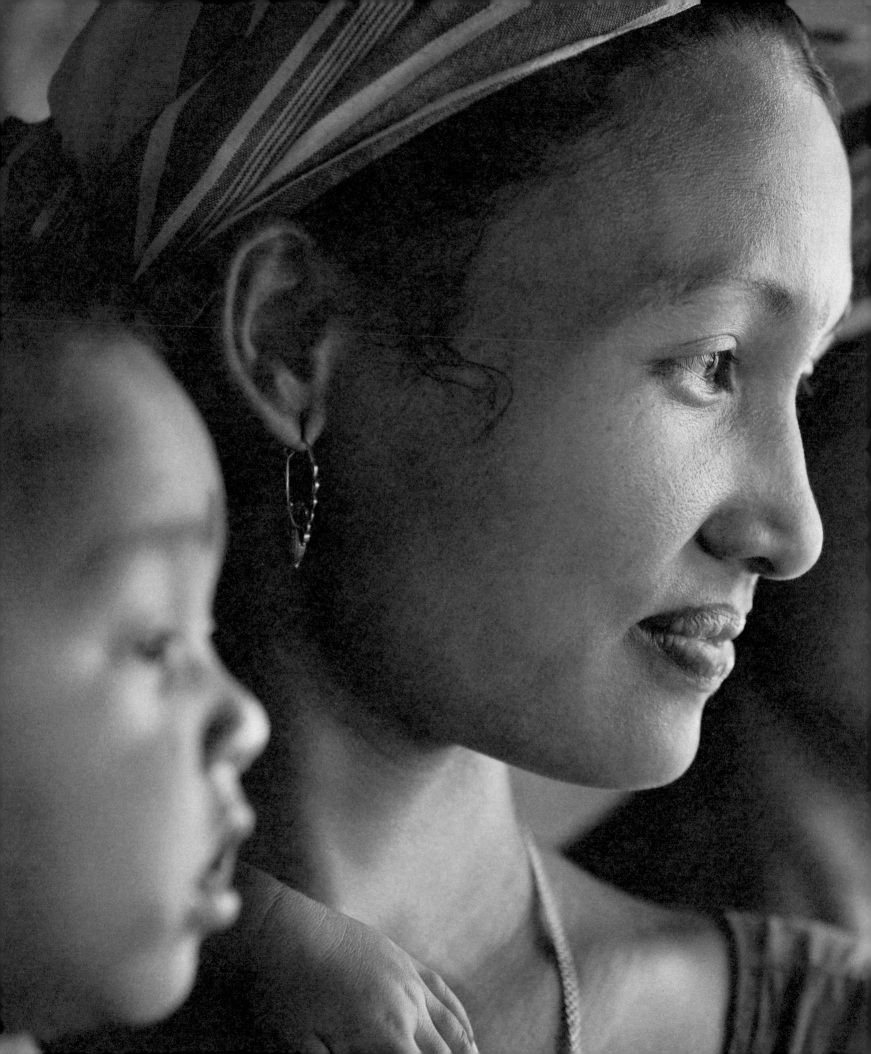

"The changing agency of women is one of the major mediators of economic and social change, and its determination as well as consequences closely relate to many of the central features of the development process."

AMARTYA SEN, *Identity and Violence*

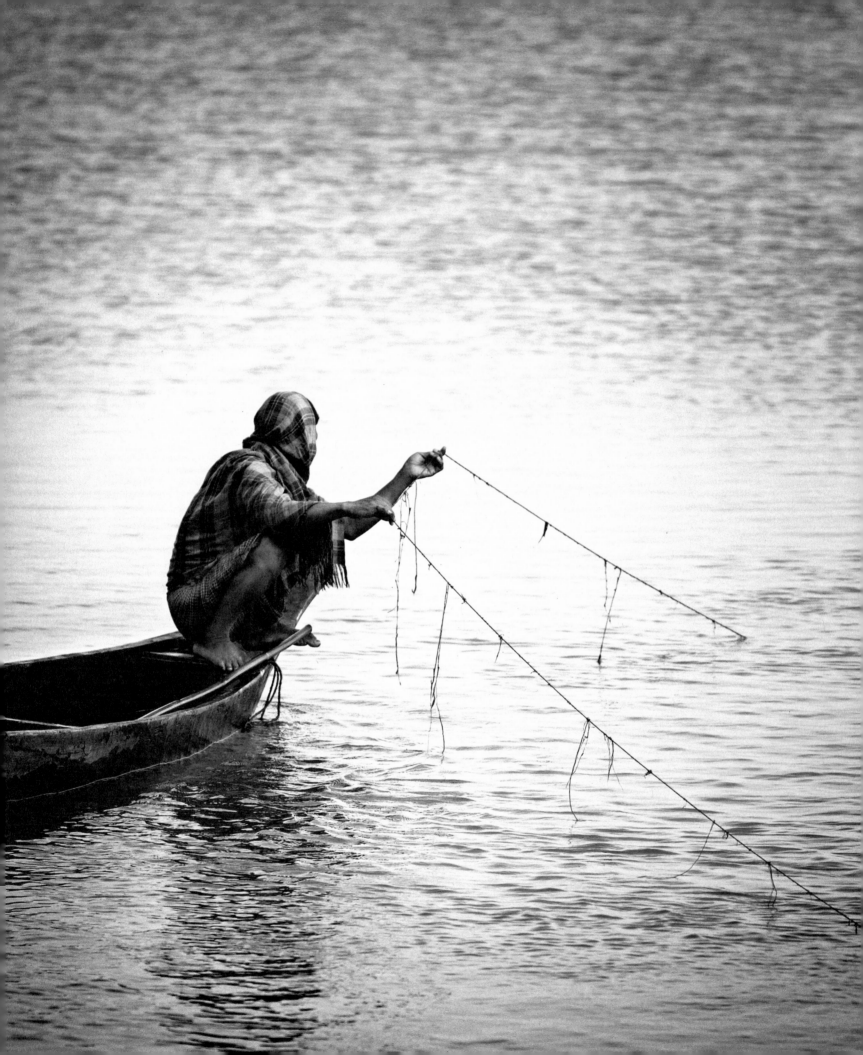

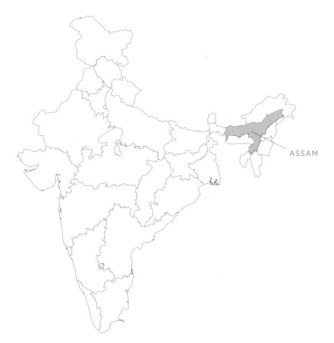

ASSAM

Energy on the
Islands of Brahmaputra

The Missing (pronounced *mishing*) tribal households live on Majuli, a large island in the Brahmaputra River in Assam, India. It is one of the largest river islands in Asia. This river and the community's tribal culture define the lives of Missing households.

The Brahmaputra provides food for the Missing, as they depend greatly on fish from the river. They also harvest driftwood from its waters for use as fuel. When I was there in April 2012, one woman in Kamala Bari village on Majuli Island told me, "It is very good wood, and you do not need a lot." Island villages on the riverbank make good use of it, also utilizing the dried stalks of a riverbank weed called *Kalmu* (*Ipomoea carnea*) in Assamese. That spring, I saw dried stalks of it piled high near the homes on Majuli.

Almost a month after that trip to Majuli, on a Sunday morning in late June, I was concerned with how those Missing villages and households that I visited were faring. *The New York Times* and *The Times of India* were reporting that the Brahmaputra had turned on its own islands and people it supports, due to a heavy monsoon in Assam and the rest of northeast India. A swollen Brahmaputra had flooded Majuli, killing many on the island and uprooting homes built on stilts, hardly an obstacle for a raging river.

Just months before, women in the villages on the riverbank were telling me about severe shortages of wood during the rainy season; collecting driftwood in the swift currents of the mighty Brahmaputra is very difficult, if not deadly, they told me. Now, with Majuli underwater, cooking is perhaps nearly impossible, with whatever dry *Kalmu* that had been stored for a rainy day now wet and useless. Another option is to bring wood from many of the river's small islands, where needly *Casuarina equisetifolia* trees grow. But how does one navigate a furious river on small boats? Surely, such ventures to bring fuelwood from these outlying islands, in small wooden boats, would be a death trap—and besides, these smaller islands were probably flooded. I was wondering how the women were managing on a flooded Majuli without access to the three significant sources of household fuel: driftwood from the river, *Kalmu* from the river banks, or the wood from *Casuarina* trees from outlying islands. Most households maintain reserves— but how long would these last?

It was evident in talking to Missing tribal households that, in knitting together energy supplies with these three different fuels, they could meet their daily energy needs and also make a rice beer they call *Apong* or *Saimod*, central to their social lives. Beyond their use for cooking, large quantities of rice and fuel are consumed in the making of *Saimod*. From the riverbank villages to the interior of Majuli, household fuel varied along a mix of the three sources mentioned above. As you went to the interior villages, it was more *Casuarina* wood and wood from local forests. On the riverbanks, it was largely *Kalmu*, fuelwood from *Casuarina*, and driftwood. What was surprising was the use of LPG stoves in many of the homes on the island.

A MORNING WITH A MISSING FAMILY

At 5:30 a.m. one April morning, Mark Katzman and I rented a ferry in Jorhat, Assam, and reached the banks of Majuli in about an hour. From there, we arrived in the Kamala Bari village on Majuli Island in less than twenty minutes by jeep to meet a Missing family. The husband works for a health promotion organization that ferries from island to island on the Brahmaputra. He is well-educated with a college degree; his wife stays home to care for all nine members of the family, including the children of her brother-in-law.

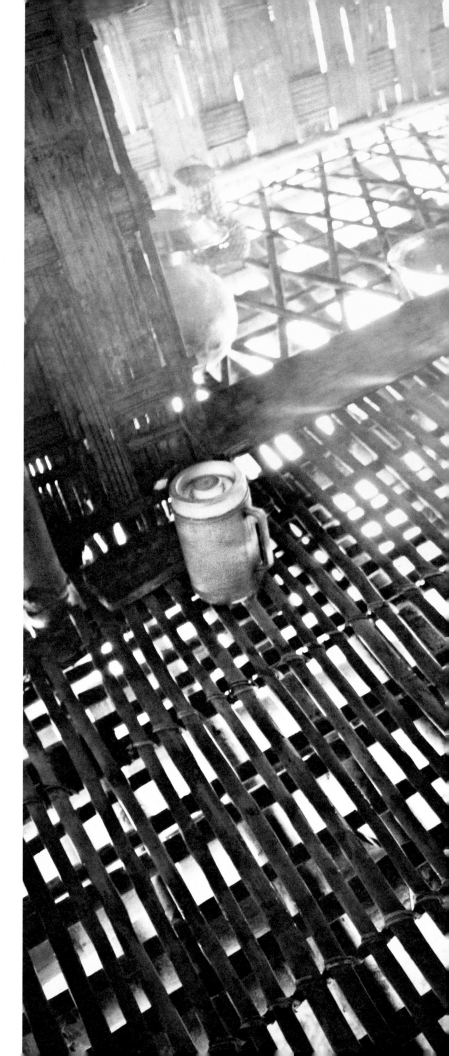

IN THE AIR

TRADITIONAL COOKSTOVE
SMOKE EXPOSURE
=
400 CIGARETTES
PER HOUR OF COOKING[1-4]

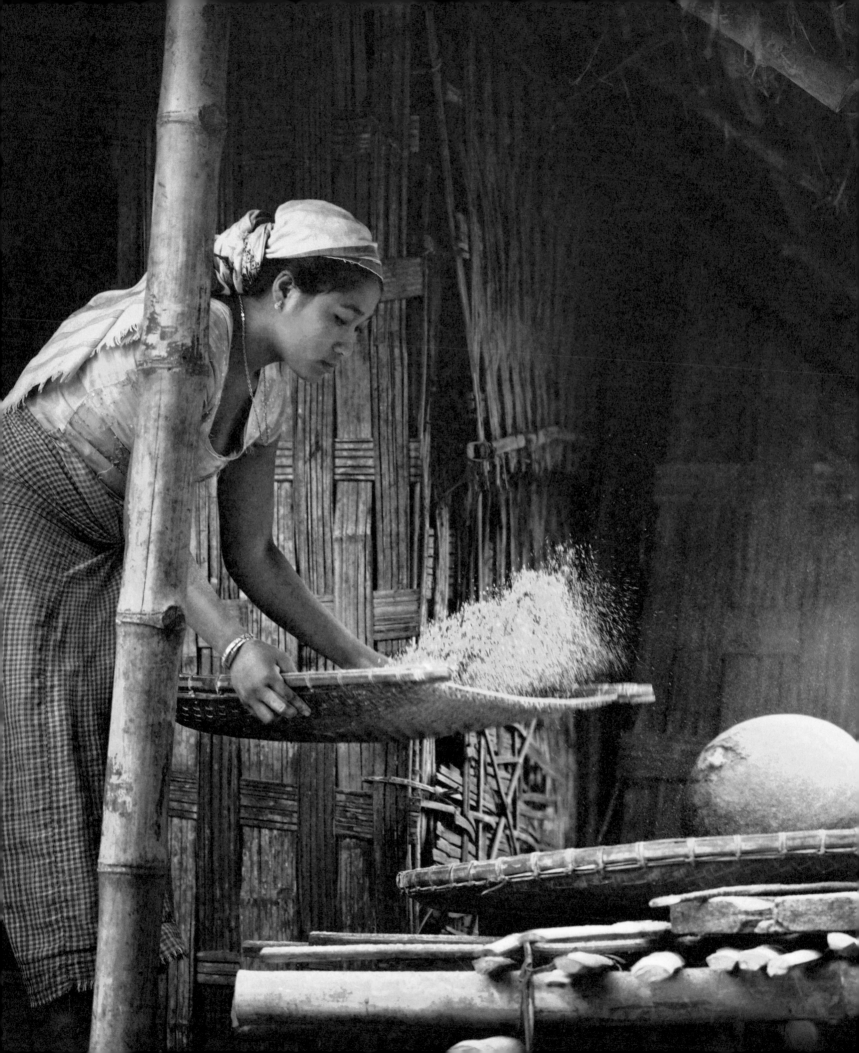

We walked into a busy morning at their home—rice was cooking for later use in brewing *Apong.* The grandmother sat around a kitchen fire, while the daughter-in-law scurried to tidy their place, which sat on stilts roughly twenty feet above the ground. She then ran into the kitchen to make tea for us, while comforting one of her daughters, who was suffering with an incessant barking cough. We began talking to the husband's sister, who told us that cooking would begin once the kids go to school, around 8:00 a.m., and continue for two and a half hours.

We received our tea in no time, clear evidence that this home had an LPG cookstove. I was eager to discuss how they made this switch and what it takes to maintain an LPG cooking stove in this village. Their answer, however, was simple: LPG was used primarily for emergencies, such as us walking into this home unexpectedly, or for a rainy day when fuelwood was scarce or too wet to burn. This family was not alone, I would learn: out of the forty-three households in this village, all but five or six had an LPG stove, yet none of them used LPG in everyday use.

This Missing household we visited purchased a month's worth of wood for about 500 rupees ($9 U.S. at the time of this writing). They considered this a bargain compared to 400 rupees for each cylinder of LPG, which would likely last two weeks if used daily. The young mother told me that it takes less driftwood to get by—only about seven to ten kilos of wood in a day. Her sister-in-law chimed in that another benefit of using driftwood was the slow and steady heat it produces. Finally, though, the family's wife—who, unsurprisingly, uses firewood to cook nearly 100% of the time—made a simple but significant statement that resonated strongly: A Missing household without a fire inside is not truly a Missing home.

HAULING WOOD FOR ALCOHOL

As mentioned briefly above, Missing households also need fuelwood to brew *Apong* or *Saimod.* In all the interior villages, the toll on a household's rice and wood quantity due to the culture of making *Apong* was enormous.

In the village of Namuni Serpai, I stopped to talk with a woman who stirred rice in her backyard in a large cauldron. Her quick calculations were as follows: it takes about two and a half hours to collect wood from a nearby forest area, and she estimated that it takes thirty kilograms of wood at a time to make *Apong* and cook regular meals for her family. One of the men, who also belonged to the Missing tribe, declared that their culture of brewing rice beer was catastrophic because of the large sums of wood deployed to brew a drink that diverted equally large sums of rice away from the food basket of the household. This was an insightful remark, indeed, and forced me to look beyond the wood required to brew, and turn my attention to food being diverted to make alcohol. Here we have an island of people spending large amounts of women's time and energy to gather wood and secure household fuel, while imposing real burdens on women to support a culture of brewing rice beer that also depletes their food grains. Powerful and deeply entrenched social norms perpetuate energy insecurity in so many ways.

On much smaller islands around Majuli, women worry about fuelwood availability, and they talk of the enormous physical strains of gathering fuelwood for household use. A primary healthcare worker that I met on one of these smaller islands—Bhakat Sapori on the Brahmaputra—spoke of women complaining of chest and shoulder pains from chopping and hauling wood from other smaller, uninhabited islands back to their homes. These women travel in small boats from their island to neighboring islands, merely to gather wood. From their description, it takes thirteen days to bring home one boatload of wood. Women from four or five households travel to islands where *Casuarina equisetifolia* is abundant. The women are joined by one man, who rows the boat.

Over two days, these women cut the necessary number of trees and leave them for drying. They return ten days later to strip the trees of the dried needle-like leaves, and prepare individual bundles roughly twenty-five to thirty kilograms in weight. Each woman, making multiple trips, then hauls one or two bundles at a time for two to three kilometers from the place of harvesting to the edge of the island where their boat and the man are waiting. Sometimes, multiple boats wait, with men ready to pack the boats with these bundles. Each woman is entitled to the same number of bundles that she is able to haul back to the boat. Large boats—long and narrow—hold approximately fifty bundles, while the smaller boats hold about thirty.

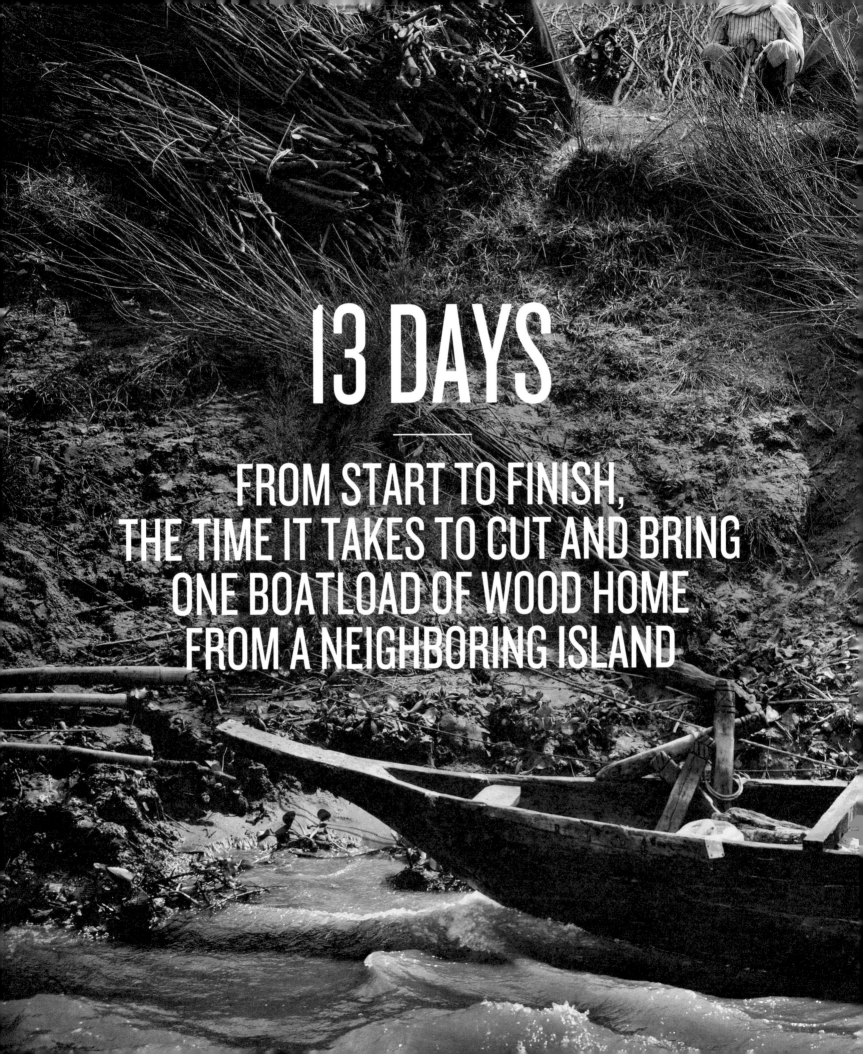

13 DAYS

FROM START TO FINISH,
THE TIME IT TAKES TO CUT AND BRING
ONE BOATLOAD OF WOOD HOME
FROM A NEIGHBORING ISLAND

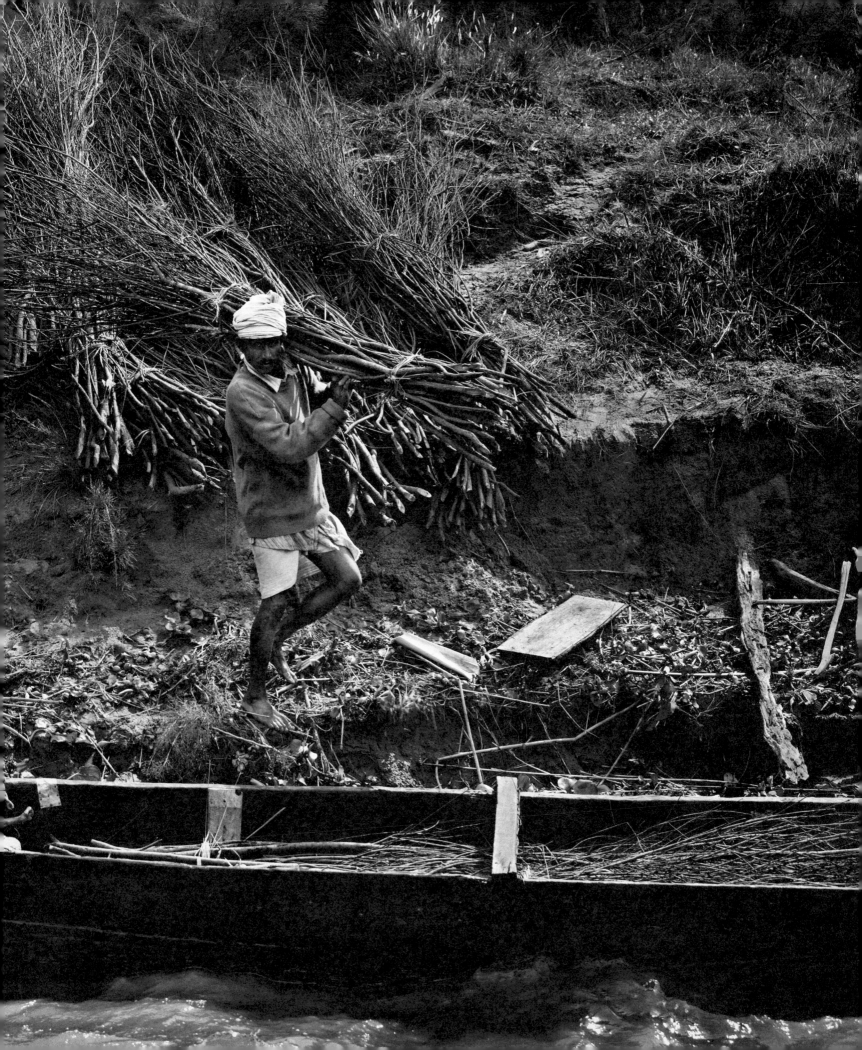

Upon returning to their home island, women then haul their bounty back to their homes. It is common to see on Majuli and on the smaller islands large stockpiles of wood bundles, sometimes up to sixty bundles, each weighing twenty-five kilograms, that women from that household have accumulated through repeated boat trips to other islands. Such is the planning, effort, and sheer physical stamina on the part of each household, particularly Missing tribal women, on these islands of Brahmaputra to keep the fires burning to feed and brew *Apong* for their families. It is their obligation and a social norm, and women, sometimes even in pregnancy, shoulder it with careful planning and mammoth effort. If not for their work, how will Bhakat Sapori, an isolated island of 225 households spread across fourteen villages, most without electricity, be able to meet daily energy needs?

Cultural and social norms are compelling, and memories of adversity are short-lived on Majuli and other islands of Brahmaputra. Missing households on Majuli will forget the misery of this recent flooding in a few short months, and return to their routines. They will go back to their riverbank and island ways on the mighty Brahmaputra. They will go back to dried stalks of *Kalmu*, much derided for its invasive and corrosive impact on local ecosystems, but an important source of fuel for Majuli villages. Dangerous currents will subside; people will collect ambling driftwood on the river. They will row their boats full of women from their island to islands of *Casuarina* wood, then cut, dry, and haul back boats full of wood for women to cook and brew. A cycle of energy-impoverished lives will continue. Smoke will billow from Missing households, and fires will burn from morning until night, providing food and comfort. Missing households without fires are not traditional. Like the woman in Kamala Bari said, "This is a traditional system; if there is no fire in the house, it is not a house. In the evening time when we pray, we need this fire. We get warmth, and the smoke helps with keeping out the mosquitoes." ❖

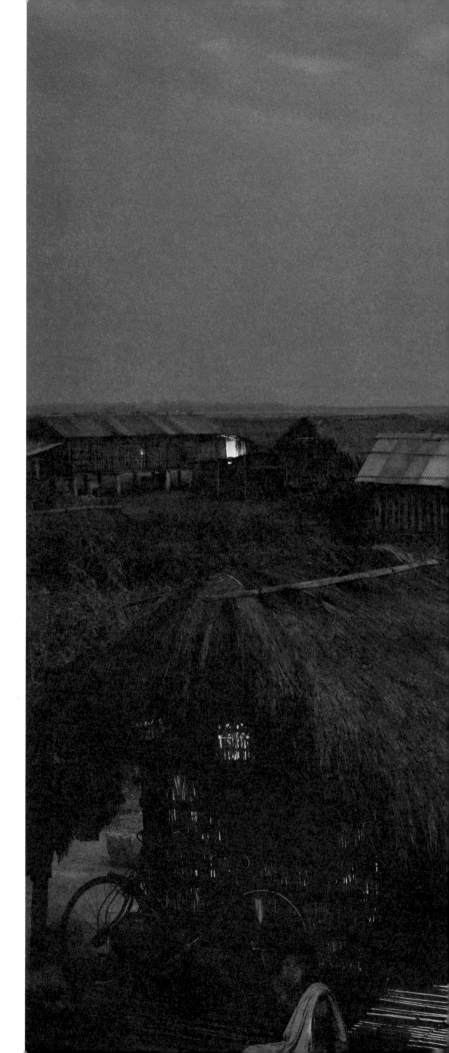

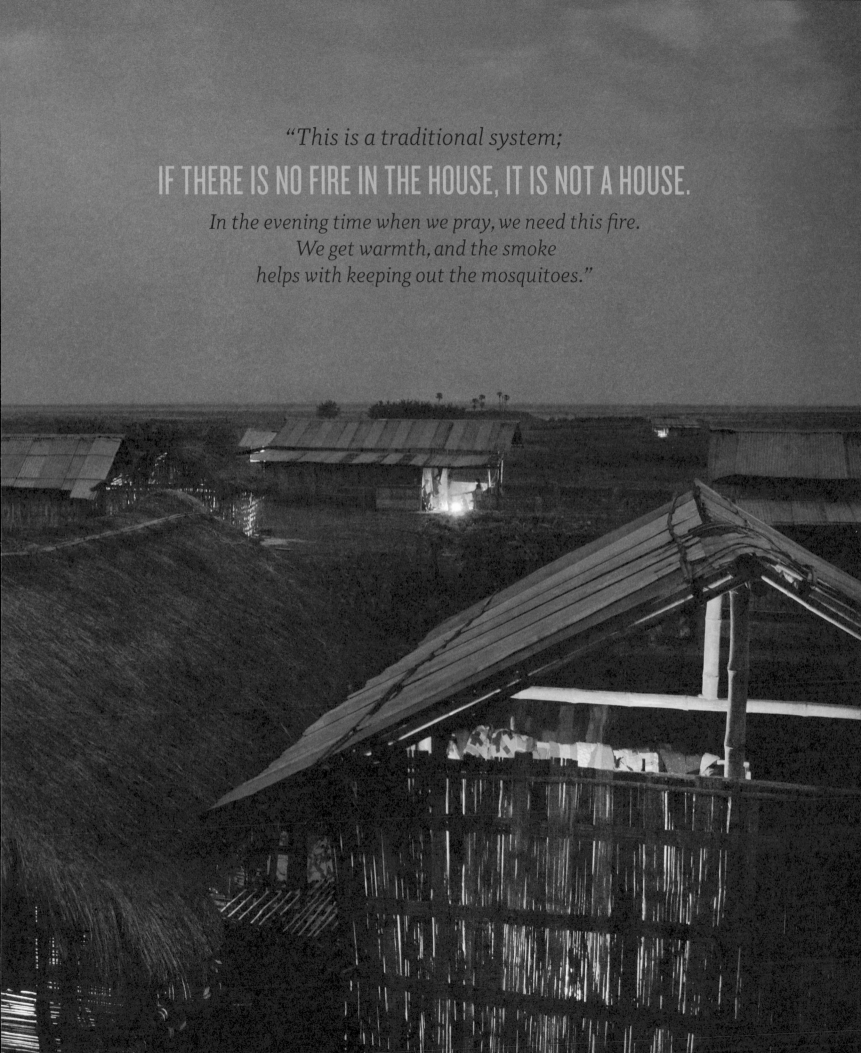

"*This is a traditional system;*
IF THERE IS NO FIRE IN THE HOUSE, IT IS NOT A HOUSE.
In the evening time when we pray, we need this fire.
We get warmth, and the smoke
helps with keeping out the mosquitoes."

Narrative Four

CAUSE & EFFECT

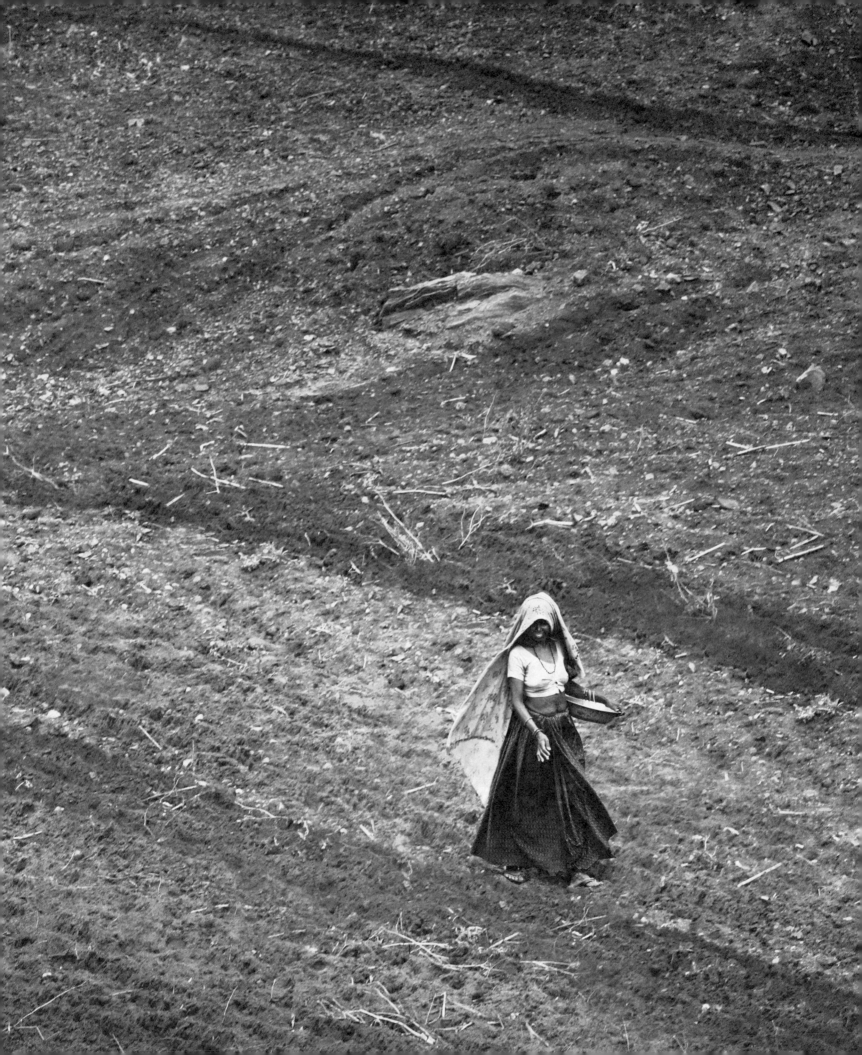

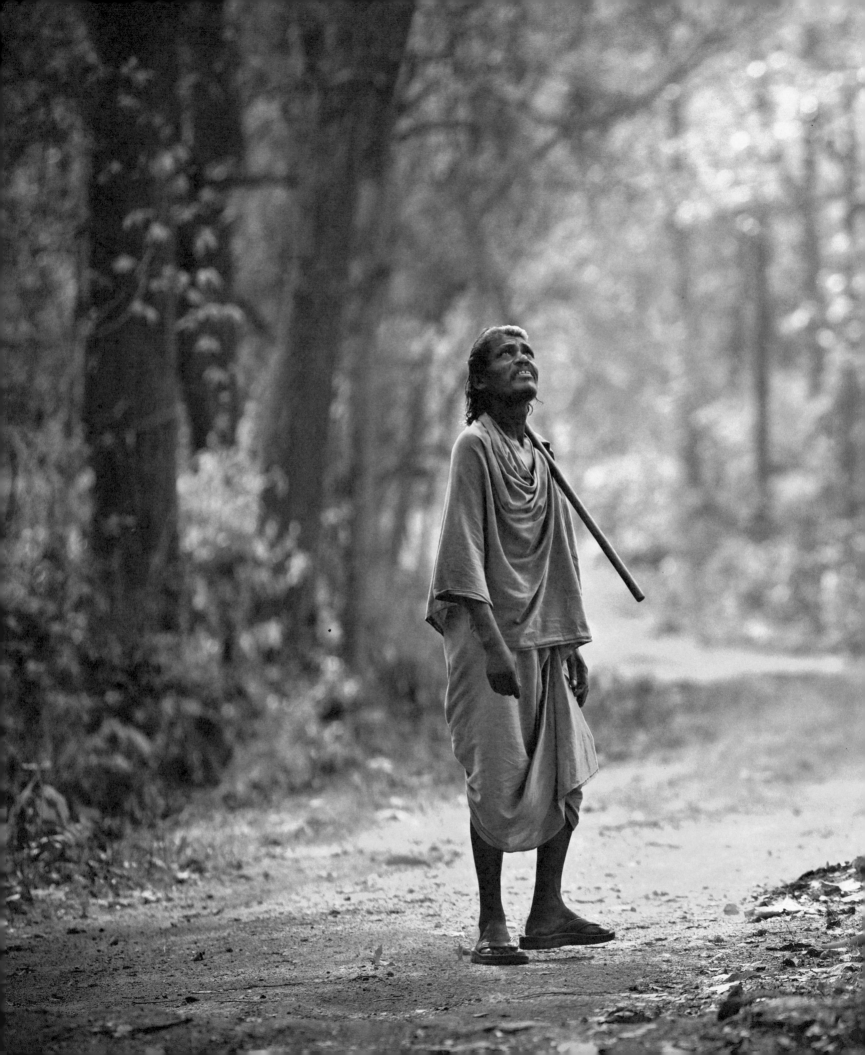

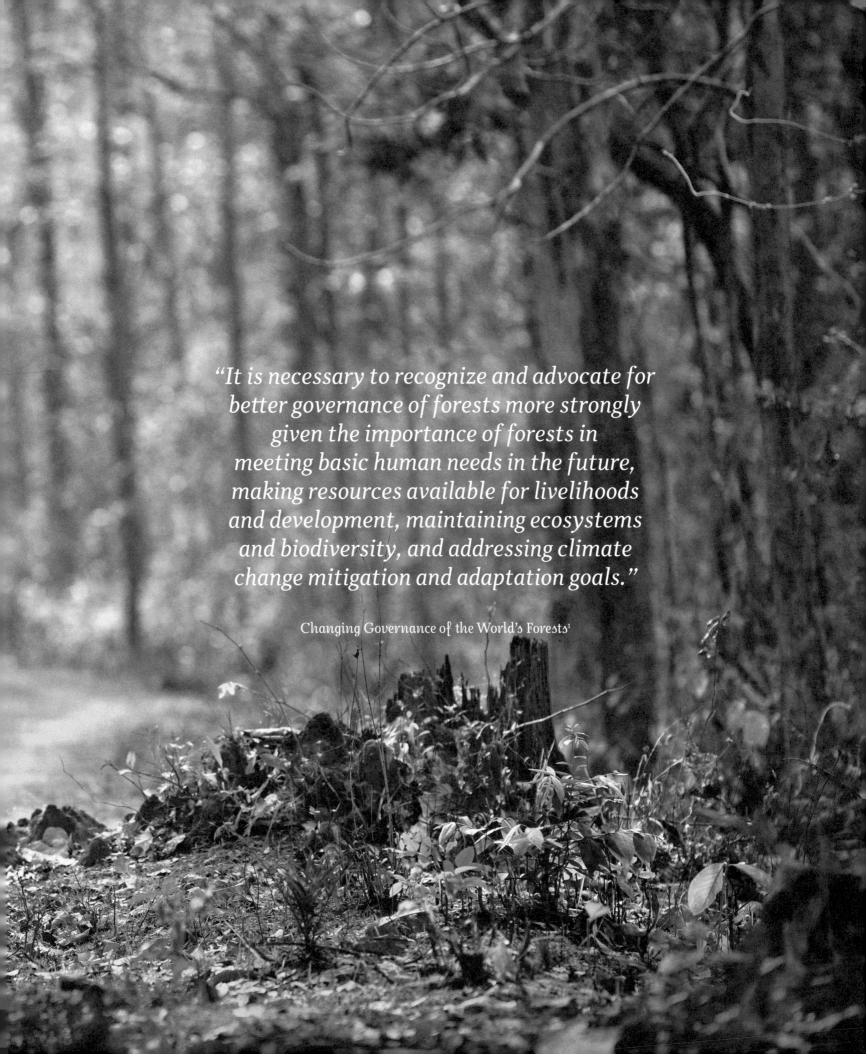

"It is necessary to recognize and advocate for better governance of forests more strongly given the importance of forests in meeting basic human needs in the future, making resources available for livelihoods and development, maintaining ecosystems and biodiversity, and addressing climate change mitigation and adaptation goals."

Changing Governance of the World's Forests[1]

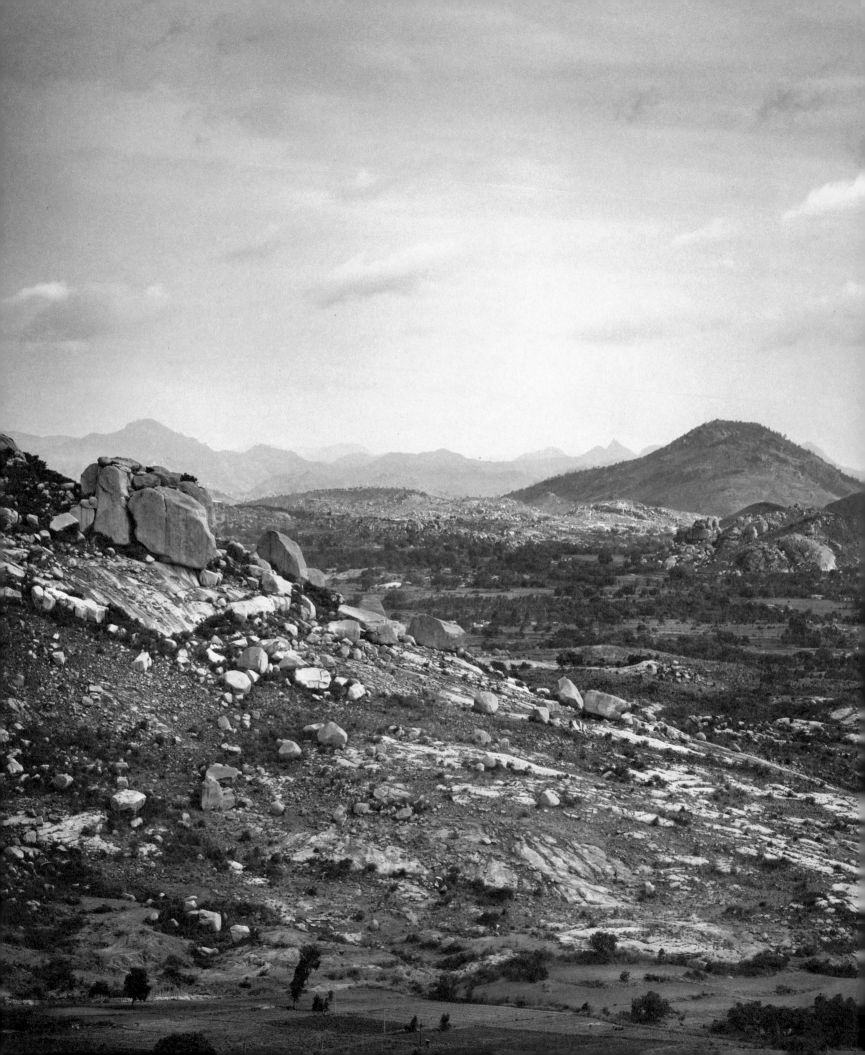

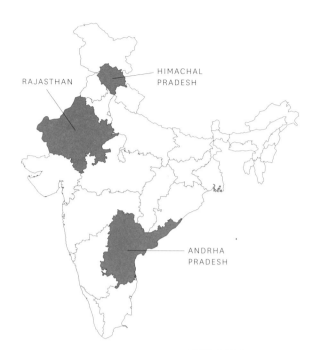

RAJASTHAN

HIMACHAL
PRADESH

ANDRHA
PRADESH

*Feedback Loops in
Andhra Pradesh and Rajasthan*

THE DYNAMIC COMPLEXITY OF AGRICULTURAL LIVELIHOODS

Risk is ubiquitous among the dryland populations of the world. The approximately 400 million people living in the drylands of India are no exception. Vulnerable to environmental risks, these communities diversify livelihoods to cushion highly variable agriculture productivity and household incomes. Policy and program interventions to reduce and buffer the poor from vulnerability to shocks are not always effective, due to the changing and dynamic nature of human and natural systems behavior. Feedback mechanisms between social, agricultural, and forest systems could produce counterintuitive impacts and reinforce the long-term vulnerability of these communities.

What is the structure of vulnerability in these complex, dynamic, and risk-prone communities, and how might they be relevant to sustained use of clean cookstoves and other clean-energy interventions? Within this narrative are some real-world cases about changing agricultural productivity and soil fertility, feedback on the trajectory of household livelihoods, and dependence on forests for fuelwood extraction to diversify livelihoods. Together they illustrate and synthesize the causal structures of vulnerability leading to counterintuitive outcomes over time that affect household livelihoods, energy decisions, natural resource conditions, and the viability of clean-energy interventions.

Over a three-year period starting in 2008, my colleagues and I partnered with the Foundation for Ecological Security (FES) in India to engage specific communities in Andhra Pradesh and Rajasthan. Our goal was to understand human and natural systems interactions with a particular emphasis on knowing more about fuelwood dependence for household energy, and to learn about their perspectives on alternative energy sources, including biogas. Our efforts in particular have been focused on communities in the dryland regions that depend on agriculture, forests, and other common lands to support their livelihoods. An important dimension of agriculture and forest interaction has to do with households that secure income and resources from forests to meet their needs routinely, and not just when farming and agriculture fail. Forests support the energy demands of the poor via firewood, water for drinking, and fodder for their animals.[2-5] Failure of agriculture and farming is due not only to sudden stresses, but also to gradual, accumulated changes in the forest ecosystems linked to tenuous household livelihoods with highly variable income, food, and energy security.

FAILING MONSOONS, DECLINING AGRICULTURE, AND SHIFTING LIVELIHOOD STRATEGIES

In 2008, with the help of FES, we gathered multiple villages from around the Madanapalle region of Andhra Pradesh to discuss their livelihood strategies. We were attempting to develop qualitative models about the problems central to villagers' livelihoods, and to determine the salient drivers of an identified problem. Villagers unanimously said that declining soil fertility is a problem that affects their livelihoods. From those meetings, and from subsequent meetings in July 2009, it became evident that certain strategic household decisions in diversifying their income streams produced changes in both long-term agricultural productivity and the productivity of forests adjacent to agricultural lands. The relevance of knowing and understanding rural livelihoods as complex and changing over time, in support of the effective dissemination and implementation of access to clean energy systems, will be evident upon my complete telling of their story.

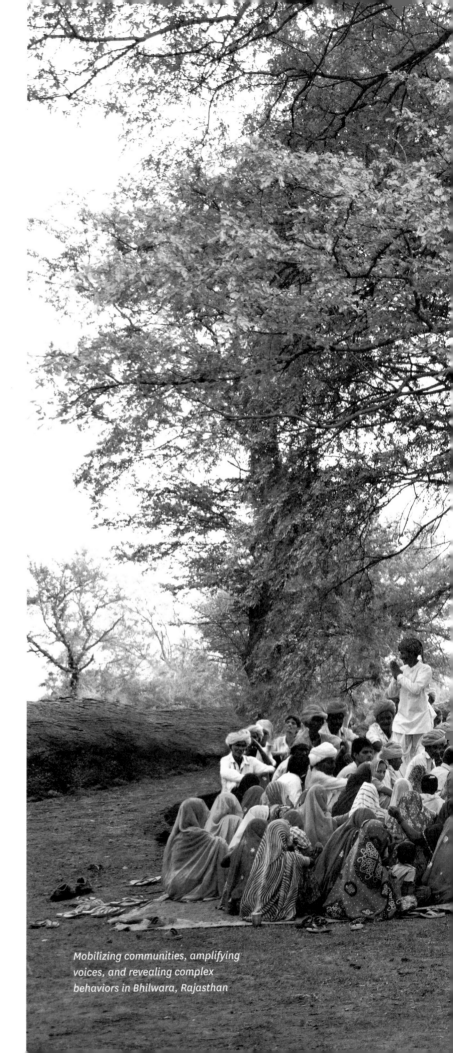

Mobilizing communities, amplifying voices, and revealing complex behaviors in Bhilwara, Rajasthan

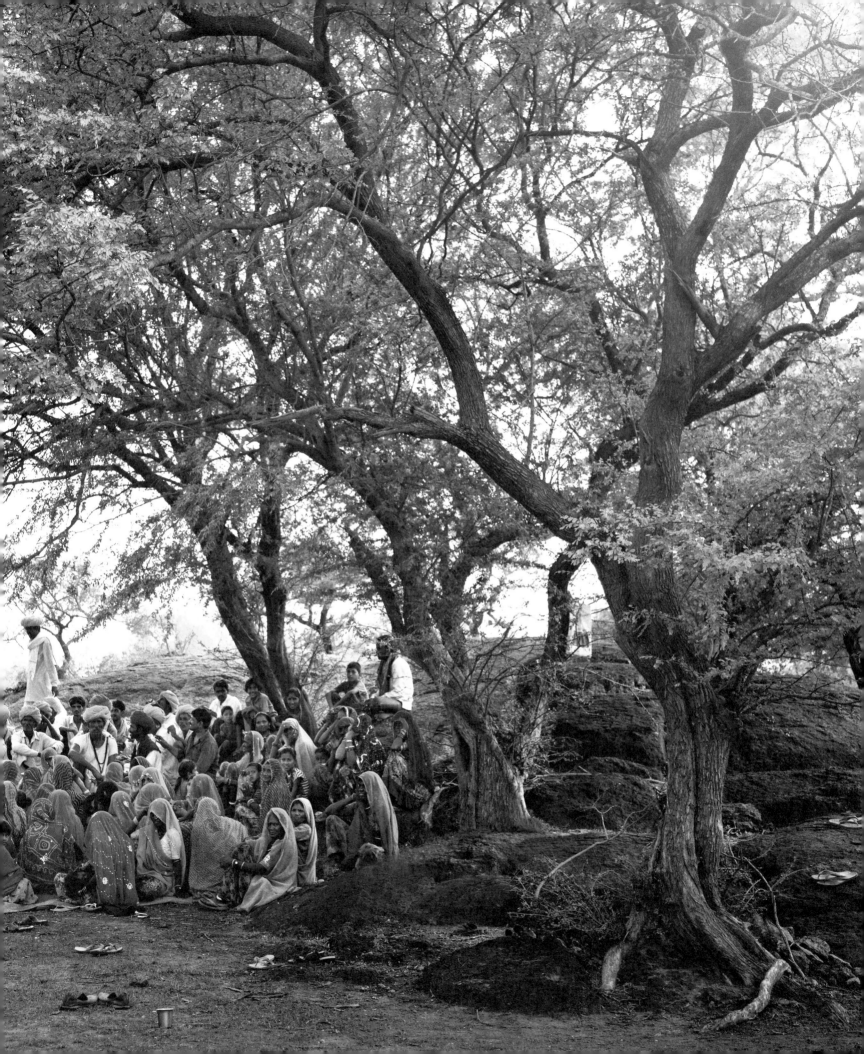

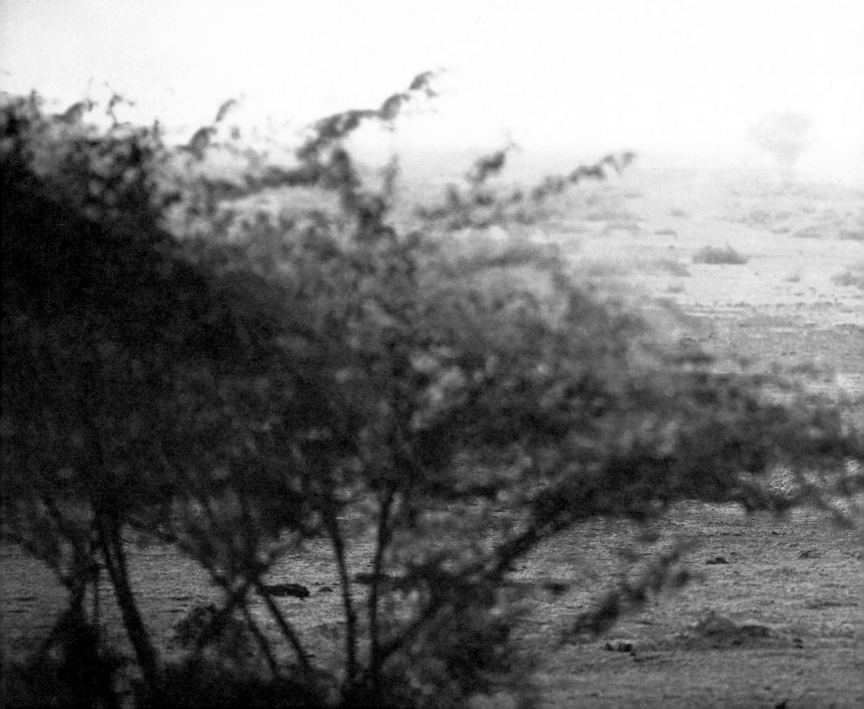

TO BUFFER AGAINST VARIABLE AGRICULTURAL INCOME, HOUSEHOLDS IN ANDHRA PRADESH SHIFTED THEIR LIVESTOCK MIX FROM NATIVE COWS TO JERSEY COWS, WHICH PRODUCE MORE MILK. THIS GENERATED THE DESIRED NEW INCOME—BUT ALSO A NEW SET OF CHALLENGES.

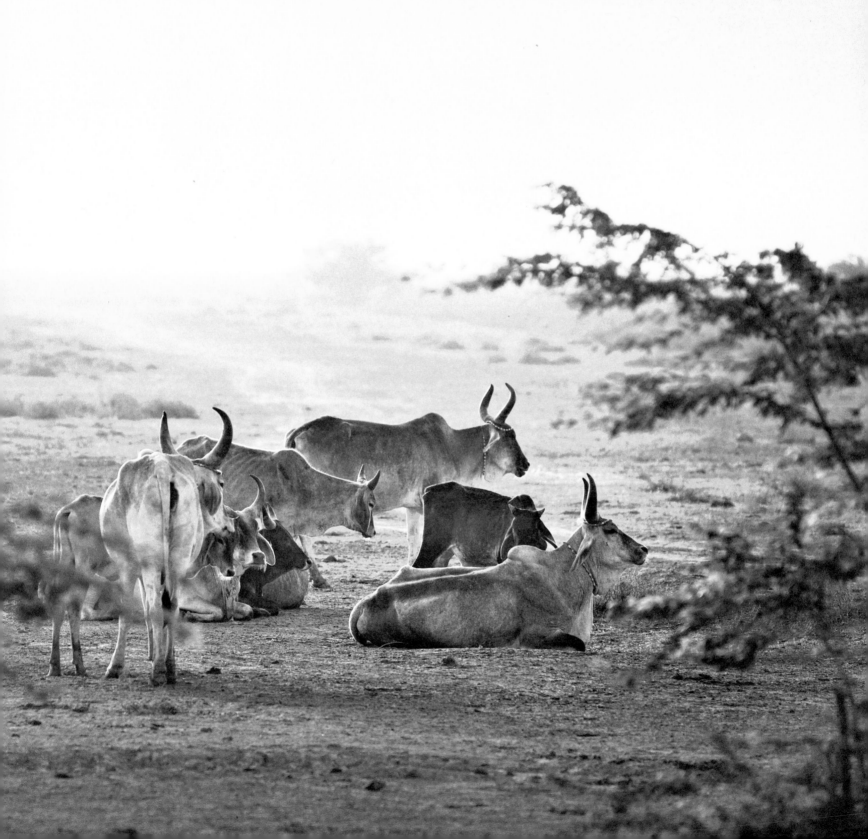

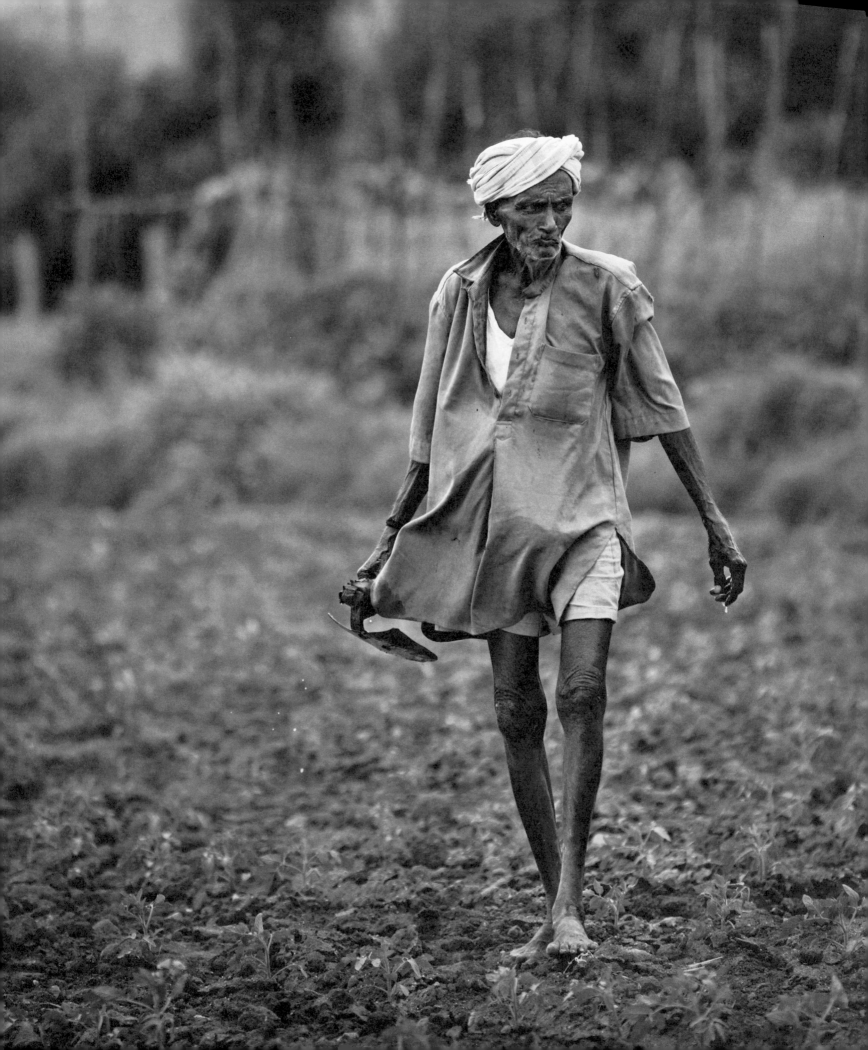

In these villages, stagnant and declining agricultural income put in motion some migration of the next generation of young people to peri-urban towns for steadier and better wages. In addition, to buffer against variable agricultural income, households shifted their livestock mix from native cows to Jersey cows, which produce more milk, to generate new income while reducing per-household livestock holdings. The shift to Jersey cows was propelled by the Andhra Pradesh government's own efforts through the Rural Livelihoods Project to promote new livestock breeds among rural households. This shift in livestock variety, by households, was also in part to reduce the physical burdens of open grazing needed for native cows, and not for Jersey cows. A local variety cow needs five kilograms of fodder and produces six liters of milk in a day, whereas a Jersey cow needs twenty kilograms of fodder and produces twenty liters of milk per day. One of the villagers equated a Jersey cow to a demon demanding large quantities of fodder to return large quantities of milk! Even with scarce fodder resources due to irregular monsoons, the increase in income from milk production sustained this shift to Jersey cows in many villages. Long dry spells, the farmers noted, also reduced fodder production from forests, a significant source of fodder in rural India.[6]

ACCUMULATED CHANGES AND UNEXPECTED OUTCOMES

Changes in agricultural livelihoods, over time, have produced other changes in the forest system. Natural pathways in the forests that were kept well-worn from livestock treading are now overgrown, with reduced open grazing as a consequence of the steady shift to Jersey cows. Well-worn cow paths, according to farmers, act as barriers to keep fires from spreading to large parts of the forest in times of drought. With reduced grazing in the forests, and overgrown paths, forest fires rage longer and spread across greater tracts of forest. Such fire damage reduced fodder production and nutrient-rich runoff from forests into adjacent agricultural lands, putting pressure on farmers to secure fodder from elsewhere; these farmers then also face declining agricultural productivity from reduced contribution of forests to soil nutrients. Shifting to Jersey cows, while increasing milk production, significantly reduced the quality of organic manure available to farmers, which led to declining returns on the farm. The result has been a weakening agricultural productivity combined with irregular monsoons that, according to farmers, have led to further declines in crop yields. Public health interventions, including clean-energy systems for better health and environment, are certain to become lower priorities when households are struggling from persistent poor agriculture productivity.

Over time, with the reduction of the absolute number of cows, farmers also noted the inability to maintain biogas units that need dung and water to produce methane used for cooking. Many who had previously shifted to biogas from wood-burning stoves could no longer depend on this alternative cleaner-burning fuel, due to lack of raw material from a decline in cow population. Their dependence on forests for wood resumed. Such feedbacks among agriculture, forests, and household decisions, mixed with well-meaning policy interventions to promote livestock to improve livelihoods, produce an unexpected impact on biogas use, fuelwood extraction, and soil fertility. These interactions underscore an underlying structure of relevant mechanisms that might explain the emergence of outcomes on the household energy front.[7]

A friend and colleague, Ashwini Chhatre from the University of Illinois, related his findings from a study of seventy villages in Himachal Pradesh that concur with these complex dynamics of rural livelihoods producing unexpected outcomes on household energy choices.[8] His study shows how there is a declining number of women going into forests to collect fuelwood with the growth in households shifting to cash crops with potential for high income. As the returns from cash crops (green peas in this example) increase, the opportunity cost of women's labor deployed in fuelwood collection increases, because labor is being diverted away from tending to green-pea production. Under such circumstances, Chhatre's field studies show women shift to other fuels—LPG or biogas—to reduce their time in fuelwood collection. His observations are illustrative of the varied interactions and interlinkages that produce both positive and adverse conditions for dissemination and implementation of clean-energy systems among rural households.

These experiences of farmers provide insights into the power of feedback effects in rural livelihoods, which are vulnerable from so many fronts. Complexity stems not only from people and natural resource interactions, but also from interactions between different categories of resources that over time transform the condition and availability of some other resource vital for people's livelihoods.

DEFORESTATION EFFECTS

When landscapes are deforested—including from fuelwood collection—the soil fertility degrades. This is because the land no longer has the input of nutrients from the decomposition of dead tree matter. Further, without the protective covering of trees, soil moisture and nutrients rapidly erode, making the soil unsuitable for most purposes.[9]

Deforested landscapes—having converted into grasslands—also reduce atmospheric water moisture. This is because grasslands have a higher "albedo" (the proportion of the incident light or radiation reflected by a surface) than forests, and thus absorb more heat; because grasslands have lower plant transpiration than forests, they release less moisture into the atmosphere.[10]

With trees, the landscape is efficient at intercepting and retaining precipitation and slowing runoff, and tree roots create large conduits in the soil that allow infiltration of water.[11] Therefore, when an ecosystem is deforested, erosion, flooding, and landslides are more common.[12, 13]

—*Tiffany Knight*

Depleting forest cover affects water runoff and recharge of groundwater table. Declining groundwater might later affect yield in agricultural output. Yet another complication in these interactions stems from differing perspectives within communities on the utility, use, and governance of resources. Complexity escalates when vital resources—livestock, agricultural productivity—are targets of state policy intervention. Governments influence community and household behavior in a particular segment of their livelihoods, but over time could produce both intended and unintended impacts on household well-being, including their household energy strategies.

CLEAN ENERGY IN REAL-WORLD SETTINGS

Our challenge is to consider clean-energy systems, while recognizing how a structure of feedback is operational in the lives of the energy poor. Household decisions to adopt, implement, and sustain clean stoves, or alternative fuels, are an outcome of interacting factors at multiple levels. To illustrate further complexity in agricultural livelihoods, consider the plight of villages in the same region that are very poor, where milk-producing livestock are absent and farmers rely on peanut crops that are monsoon-dependent.

Such communities knit together household incomes derived from growing a peanut crop and fuelwood extraction from neighboring forests to supply outlying towns within five kilometers. Households in these villages depend on agriculture and wage labor as their primary source of income, and sell fuelwood, fruits, and flowers as a secondary endeavor. Due to small land holdings (2.8 acres per household) and low productivity, annual income from agriculture is approximately 8,000 rupees ($174 U.S. in 2009), which is insufficient to support a five-member household. A quarter of the households are landless, depending on the daily wages and sale of non-timber forest products (NTFP) throughout the year. Supplementary income from forests and wage labor is critical for sustaining household livelihoods, regardless of the size of landholding. Further, intermittent drought since 2002 has forced the sale of cattle, sheep, and goats due to shortages in fodder and water. Only a small proportion of the farmers in these villages has irrigation to realize better crop yields from their small land holdings. Erratic rainfall patterns have limited the success of agriculture as the dominant livelihood strategy. This has placed added pressure on the forest, as households rely on selling fuelwood not only for supplementary income but also as a primary source of income.

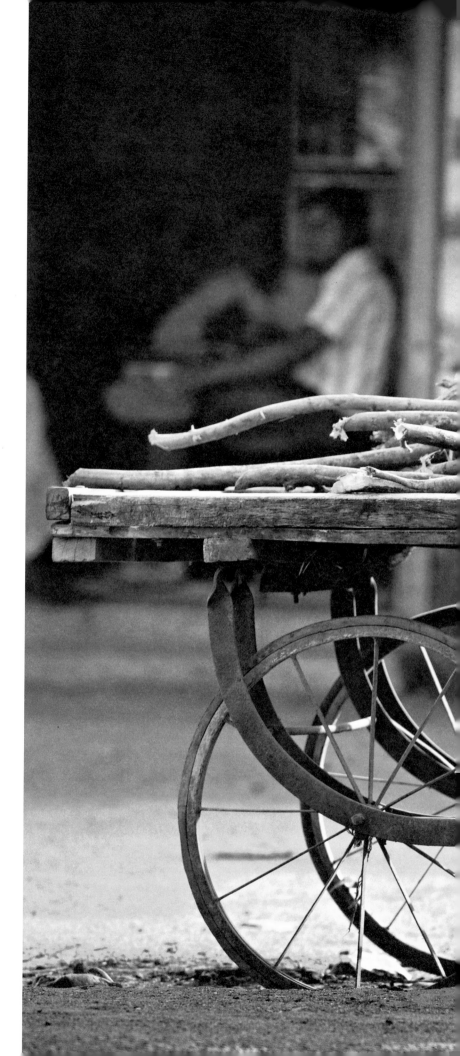

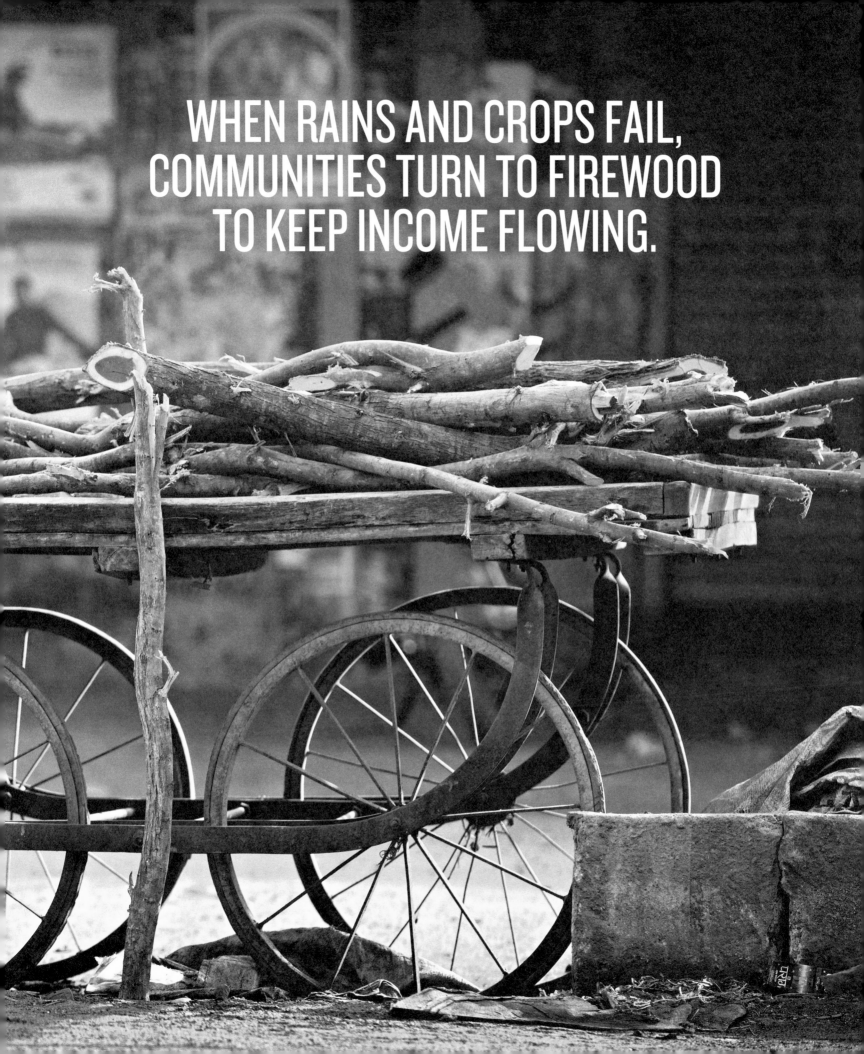

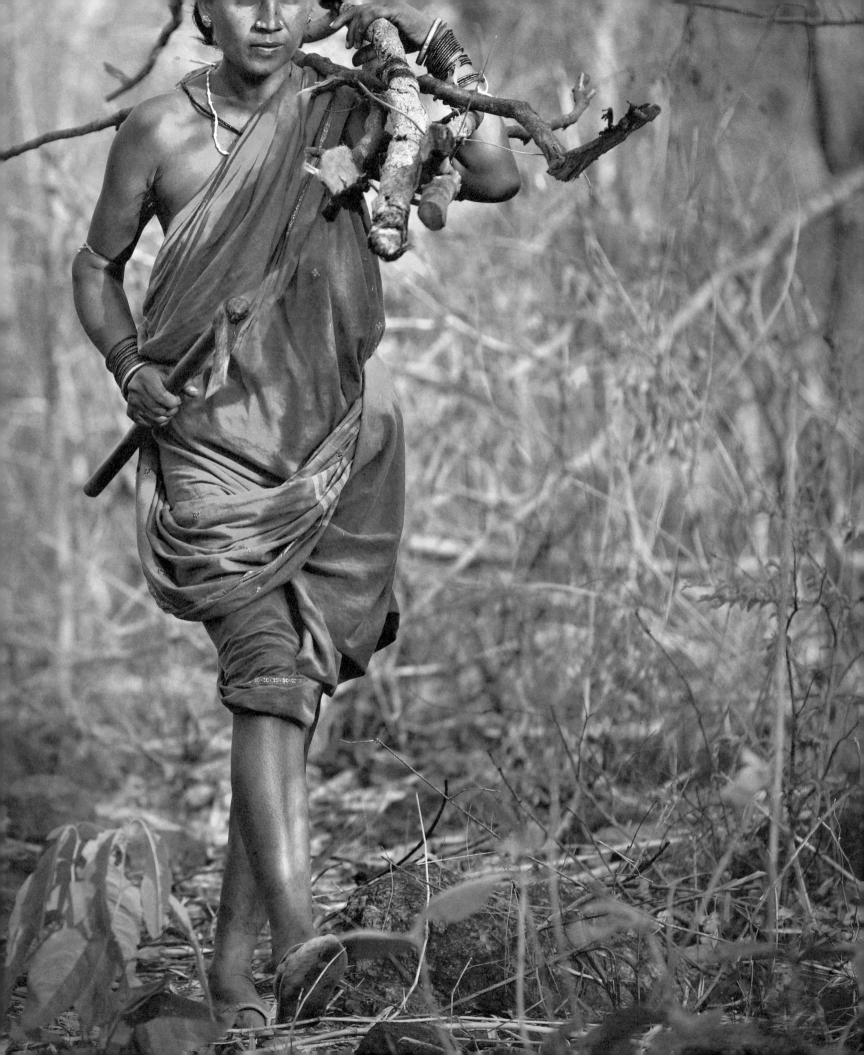

In 2009, in the middle of a severe drought, walking into such villages, all one could see were large bundles, six feet in length, stacked by the sides of homes everywhere. Crops were on the verge of failing; households had invested in seeds and planted them in anticipation of monsoons.

There was no monsoon. The sown peanuts did not germinate, crops had failed, and the only source of income was to sell fuelwood to neighboring towns.

In outlying peri-urban towns, households were in the habit of occasionally cooking with LPG, or on kerosene stoves, while also using wood. Women would extract fuel daily to make 60 rupees per bundle. They also had other unexpected burdens of paying back loans they received from the government through a very popular self-help group loan program. The program requires women, approximately ten or so, to form a group to start pooling funds every month. Once the pooled sum reaches a certain level, the government matches that amount in a loan to the self-help group. With this leveraged fund, the women invest in a variety of productive ventures, including buying seed and fertilizer.

Many women in this village, adjacent to the Sadhukonda Forest Reserve in Madanapalle, had been a part of groups that received loans, and invested those funds in buying peanut seed. Monthly loan repayments and the failed crops had a feedback effect on increased fuelwood collection for income in this village. Women were collecting good fuelwood, some for their own use, but mostly for selling. Again, tenuous livelihoods make for a complex set of conditions that modify household priorities or push them into transitory states where a stable set of priorities and livelihood trajectories are untenable. Women under such conditions adapt to using more abundantly available invasive plant and tree species, both for household energy and as a way of reserving better-quality fuelwood for income through selling. Moreover, under such conditions, households might revert back to tried-and-tested practices that require little attention, such as relying on traditional stoves, putting aside biogas or LPG systems that they might have adopted. New energy systems might be abandoned, but they might take up mobile phones to connect with outlying labor markets to engage in daily migration for wage labor.

Such are the challenges that confront improved cookstoves, or biogas, or other clean-energy systems in the context of complex agricultural livelihoods of the 3 billion people who are energy insecure. Dryland communities, whether in Andhra Pradesh, Madhya Pradesh, or Rajasthan, are vulnerable to droughts and other environmental shocks, leading to failed crops, reduced fodder, and loss of income, further compounding the burdens of prior household debt. The vulnerability of communities and households, and their ability to cope, are pertinent and could become pivotal in enabling or undermining efforts to provide clean, cost-effective energy systems for the poor. Sustained use and disuse of cleaner fuels and stoves over time, as is evident from community discussions, are an outcome of the flux in livelihoods from myriad interlinkages at multiple scales.

Feedback between various systems central to the rural poor is salient not just for implementing clean-energy systems but for other interventions to improve the lives of 160 million households in India that are energy impoverished. These millions of households are embedded in social and economic structures of rural India that confer certain resource endowments and entitlements by virtue of their social and economic position in these communities. A keen focus on social and livelihood dynamics is therefore pivotal for dissemination and implementation of clean-energy systems. Farmer narratives from Andhra Pradesh and elsewhere provide ample evidence of how such dynamics complicate the scenario for important and urgently needed clean-energy systems. The impact of interventions, including efforts to shift to new fuels or energy systems, will have differentiated outcomes as a function of households' access to other resources, endowments, and institutions of power.

Jesse C. Ribot, a geographer at the University of Illinois, put it this way in a 2009 World Bank monograph: "These different outcomes are the result of place-based social and political-economic circumstances. The inability to manage stresses does not fall from the sky. It is produced by on-the-ground social inequality; unequal access to resources; poverty; poor infrastructure; lack of representation...."[14]

Therefore, the dynamics within human social systems and other systems, as well as the relationships across them, are complex and nonlinear, and have multiple interacting feedback mechanisms.[15]

On the next spread, you will see the second of this book's two causal maps, which illustrates these feedbacks in more visual detail than the first model.

LOOPS & ARROWS

A DEEPER LOOK AT THE FEEDBACK MECHANISMS AT PLAY

For this causal map, colors differentiate the feedback mechanisms involved in energy systems used by the poor. Some background about each section:

R1: Green arrows represent feedback mechanisms related to demographic changes in people and livestock in rural Andhra Pradesh, processes that began twenty to twenty-five years ago.

R2: Red arrows denote feedback mechanisms between forest and livestock systems, tracing the linkages from livestock changes to forest biodiversity and back to influences on native livestock.

B1: Blue arrows show how agriculture production and income drive investments in agriculture, the acquisition and payment of loans, and their relation to diversification of income streams.

R3: These yellow arrows explain the feedback mechanism of communities, the opportunity cost of depending on fuelwood, and their consequences for using clean-energy systems. Starting from fuelwood extraction, this loop traces the links to forest biodiversity and to impacts on nutrient recycling into agricultural lands, soil fertility, agricultural productivity, and more, ultimately back to an influence on forest biodiversity.

R4: Pink arrows illustrate that forest biodiversity, as it is maintained or increased, will keep invasive plant and tree species at bay. When invasive species make inroads into a forest, forest biodiversity declines.

A **plus sign** indicates that two factors move in parallel ways—when one goes up or down, the other does the same. For example, when there is no cost to spending long hours collecting wood, there also will be less interest in shifting away from traditional wood burning to cleaner energy systems.

A **negative sign** on a causal link between two factors means that these factors are moving in opposite directions. When one factor increases, the related factor decreases. When people increasingly use clean-energy systems, for instance, their fuelwood extraction will decrease.

CASE IN POINT: A LOOK AT R3

For the story of reinforcing loop R3, let's begin with fuelwood extraction by millions of households. Over time, fuelwood extraction from forests leads to a decline in forest biodiversity. As forest biodiversity declines, there is an associated decline in the nutrient-rich runoff from forests that contributes to soil fertility. Declining soil fertility in surrounding agricultural lands, in time, puts a downward pressure on agricultural productivity. As agricultural output declines, so does income of households. When income from agriculture is low, the opportunity cost to a household in spending more time collecting wood will also be low. Under such conditions, households are also less likely to shift to clean-energy systems built on cleaner fuels or efficient combustion, because the cost of shifting is great. A reluctance to shift continues a pattern of fuelwood extraction that reinforces already declining forest biodiversity. To be sure, this reinforcing mechanism could easily work in the opposite direction, where declining fuelwood extraction leads to increasing forest biodiversity and so on. It is important to recognize that the numerous feedback mechanisms represented in the figure are interlinked, and over time, some mechanisms become more dominant than others in driving the use of clean-energy systems. But it is important to recognize that the uptake of clean-energy systems is part of a complex set of interrelated feedback structures. ✿

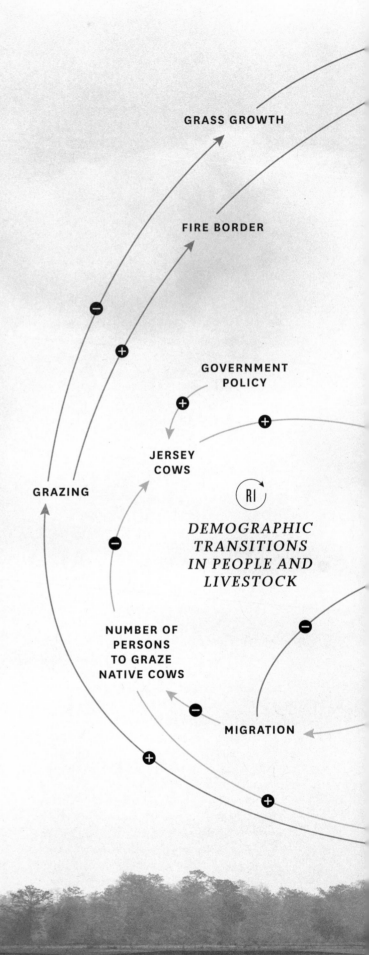

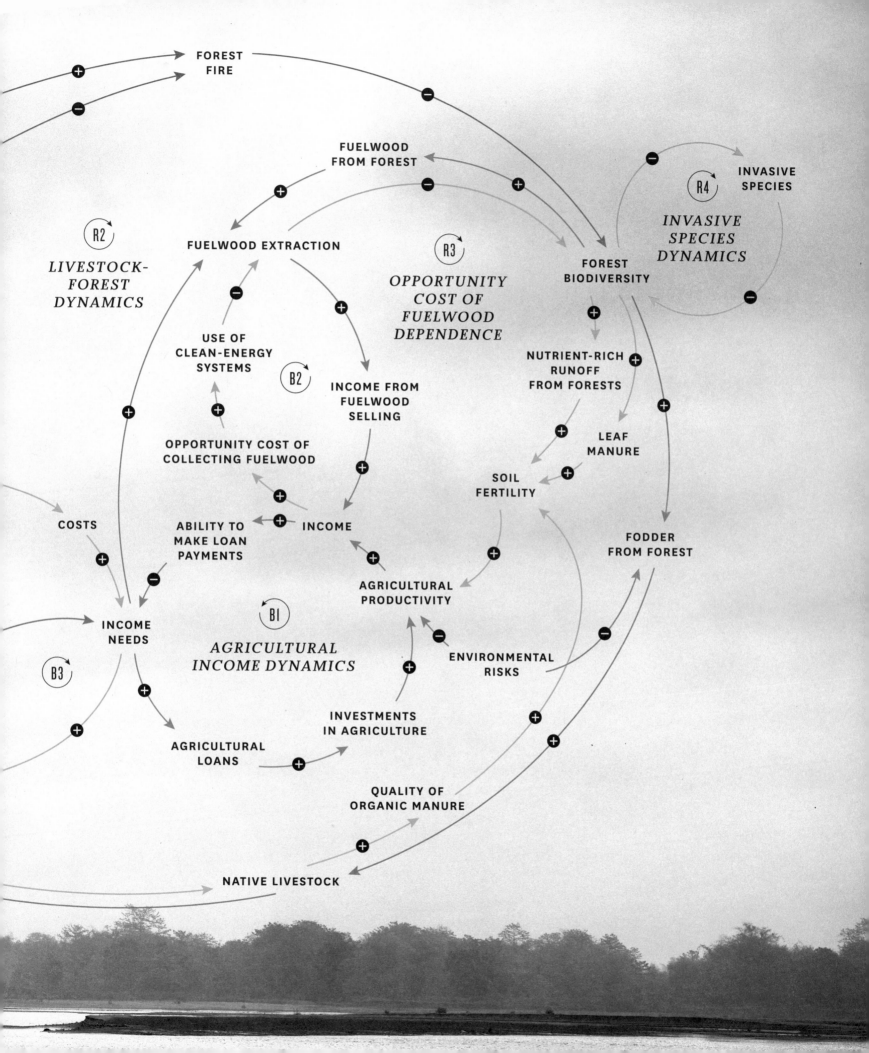

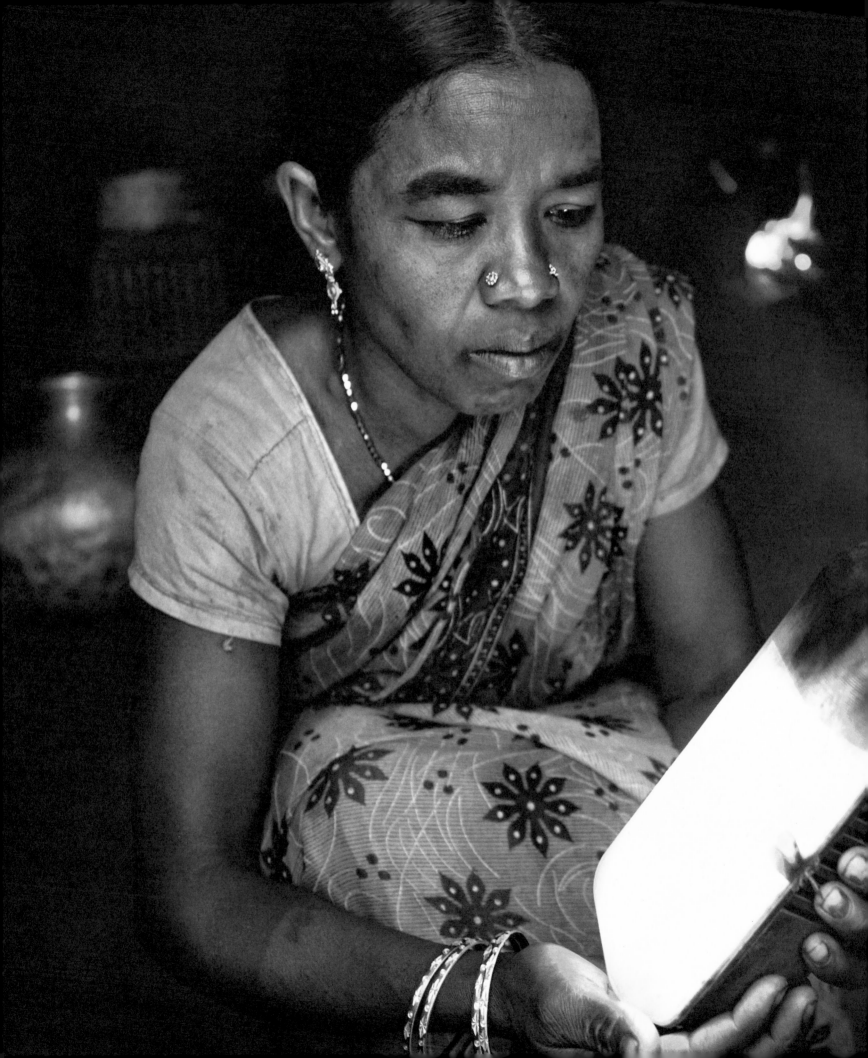

Narrative Five

SEARCHING FOR AGENCY

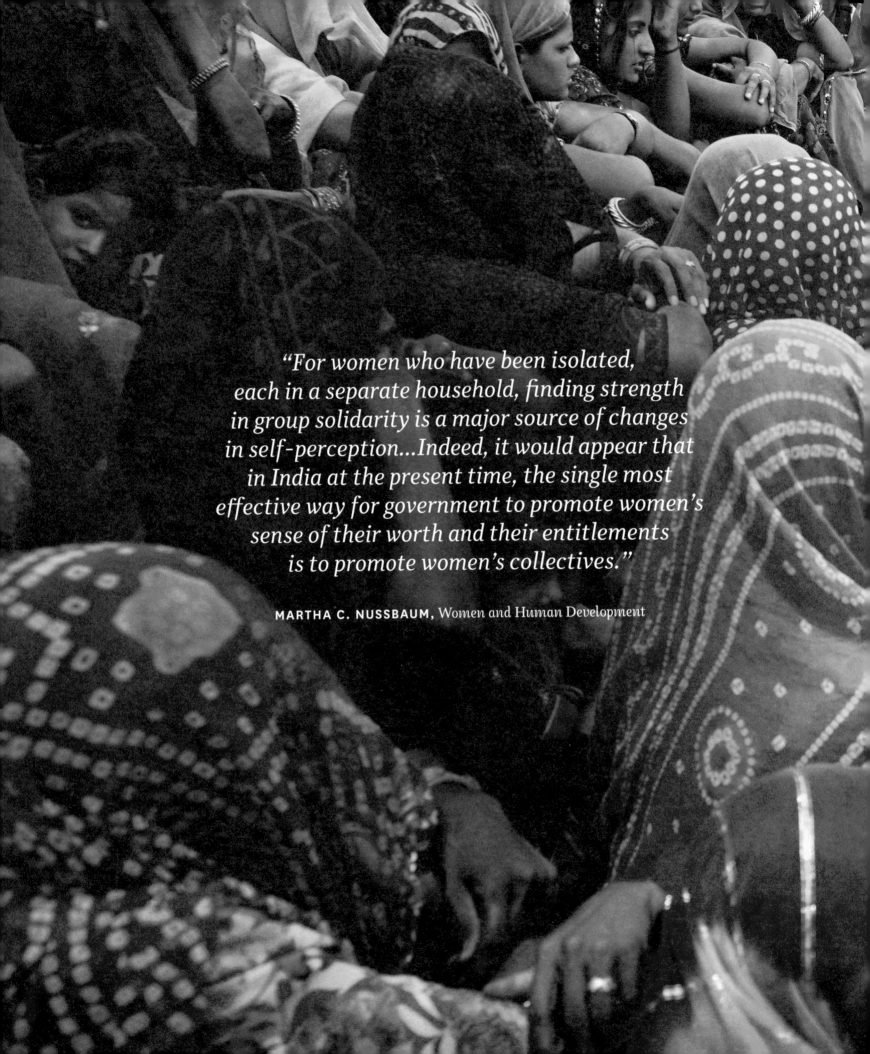

"*For women who have been isolated, each in a separate household, finding strength in group solidarity is a major source of changes in self-perception...Indeed, it would appear that in India at the present time, the single most effective way for government to promote women's sense of their worth and their entitlements is to promote women's collectives.*"

MARTHA C. NUSSBAUM, *Women and Human Development*

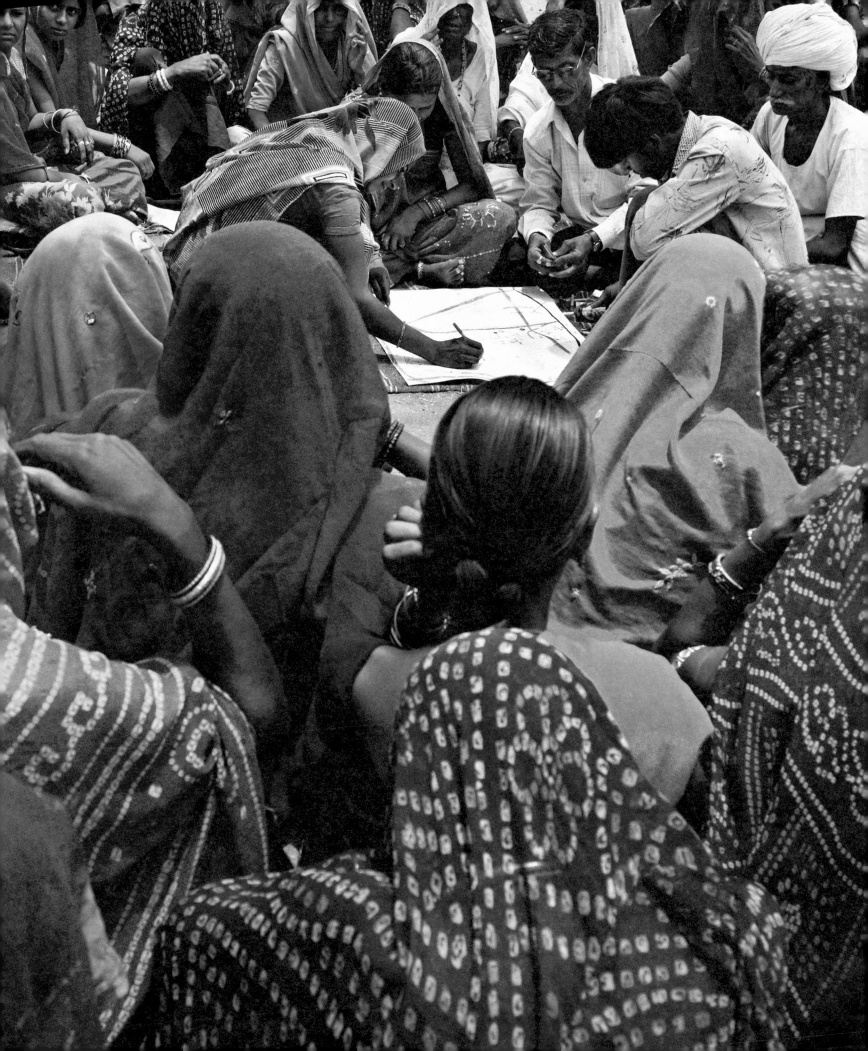

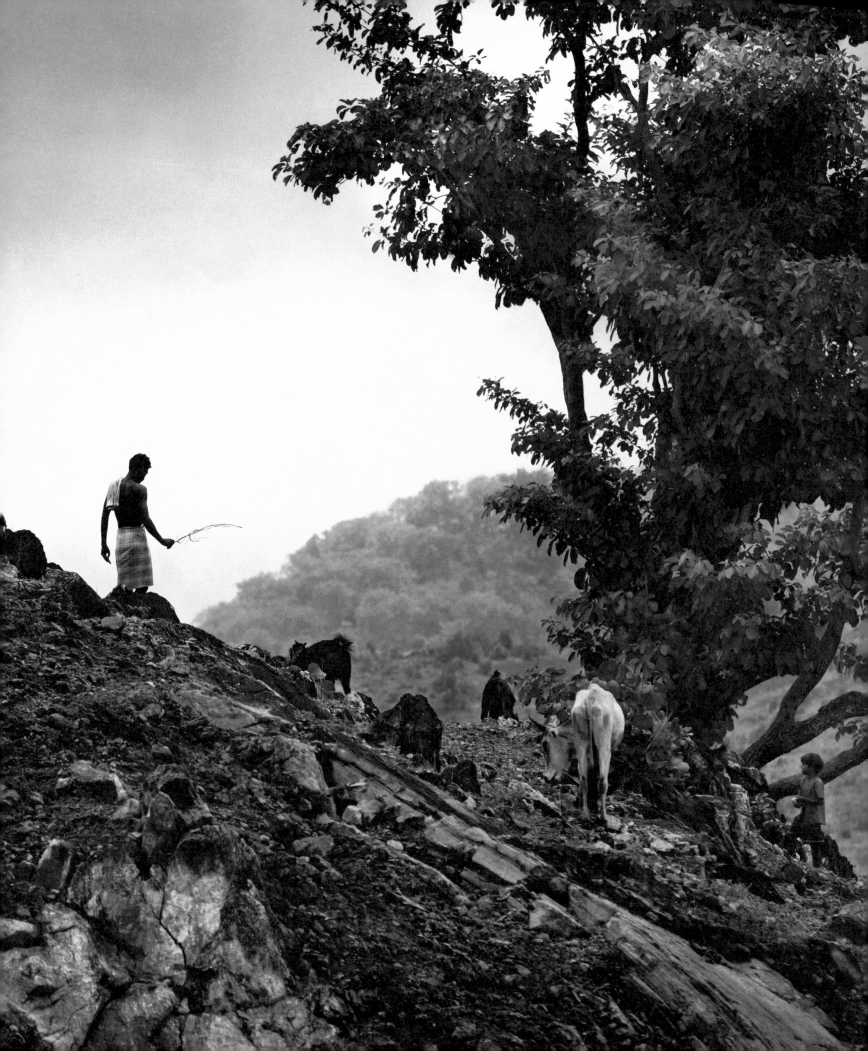

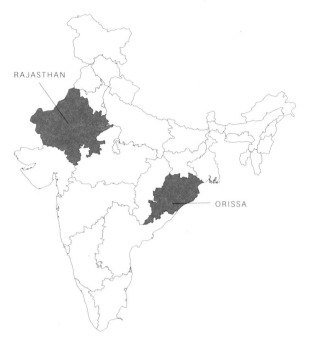

RAJASTHAN

ORISSA

*The Power of People
and Communities*

INNOVATING, ADOPTING, AND ABANDONING

Depleted forests—combined with soil erosion—have taken a toll on forest health, agricultural systems, and the sustainability of households in the Aravalli hill range of Rajasthan. It does not take much to notice the severe ecological stress and the adverse impact on human lives.

People, nevertheless, persist in these hills, relying on unproductive agriculture and ecosystems for food and energy. Unexpectedly, in the midst of threadbare living, they also adopt and invest in new technologies that they consider necessary.

In 2011, I was at the home of a 28-year-old man who owned a very small amount of farmland; he earned his income from working in a plant nursery for a local nongovernmental organization. When I walked up to his house in the village of Rawach in Udaipur district, I noticed two small solar panels—the size of a notepad, but square in shape—on his rooftop. A woman, presumably his wife, was collecting yard waste and preparing to cook on a traditional stove. Assuming that the solar panels were to power a light bulb, I inquired about their use.

The man related three surprising facts.

First, the purpose of the two solar panels was to charge his mobile phone, and not to power a light bulb as I had assumed.

Second, he was not given these panels, but purchased them for 600 rupees total ($14 U.S. at the time of the conversation), a handsome amount for a poor farmer in a removed habitation of the Aravalli hills of Udaipur district in Rajasthan, India.

And third, he was able to purchase the panels from a general store in Gogunda, a crossroads town that is some distance away from his habitation in the hills. When I further inquired about this, he added that not one, but *two* general purpose stores in Gogunda supply these solar panels for charging a mobile phone.

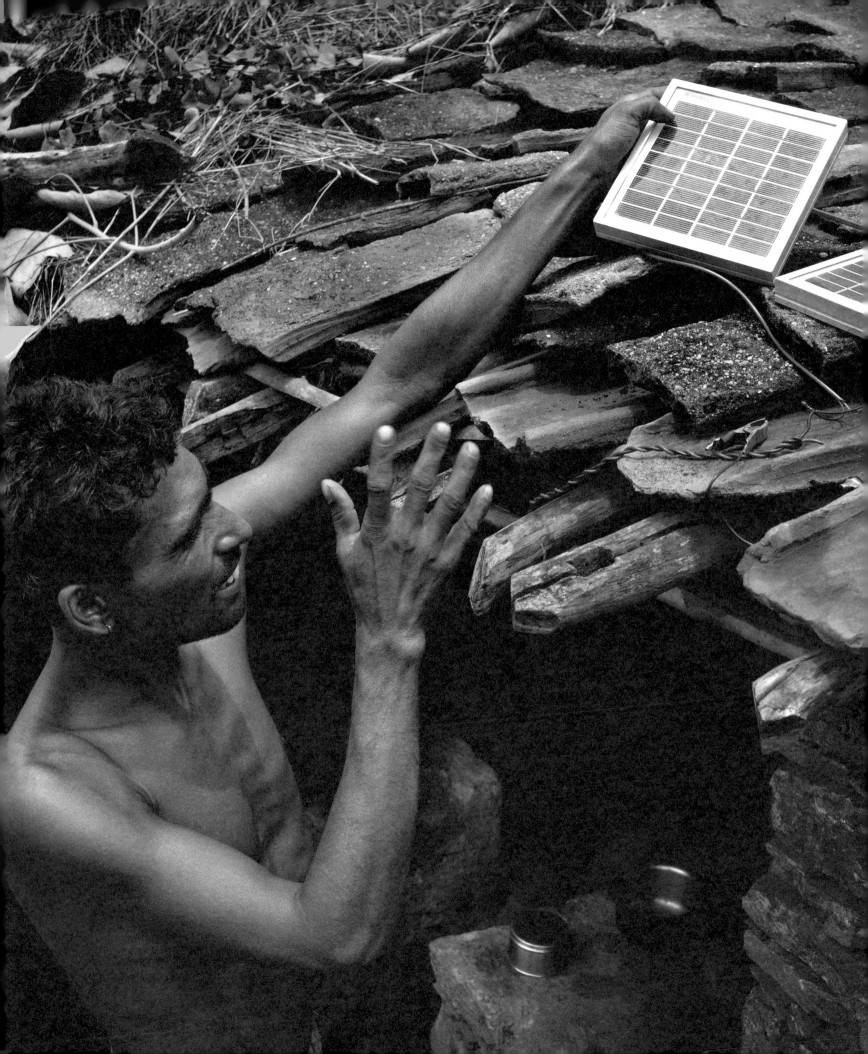

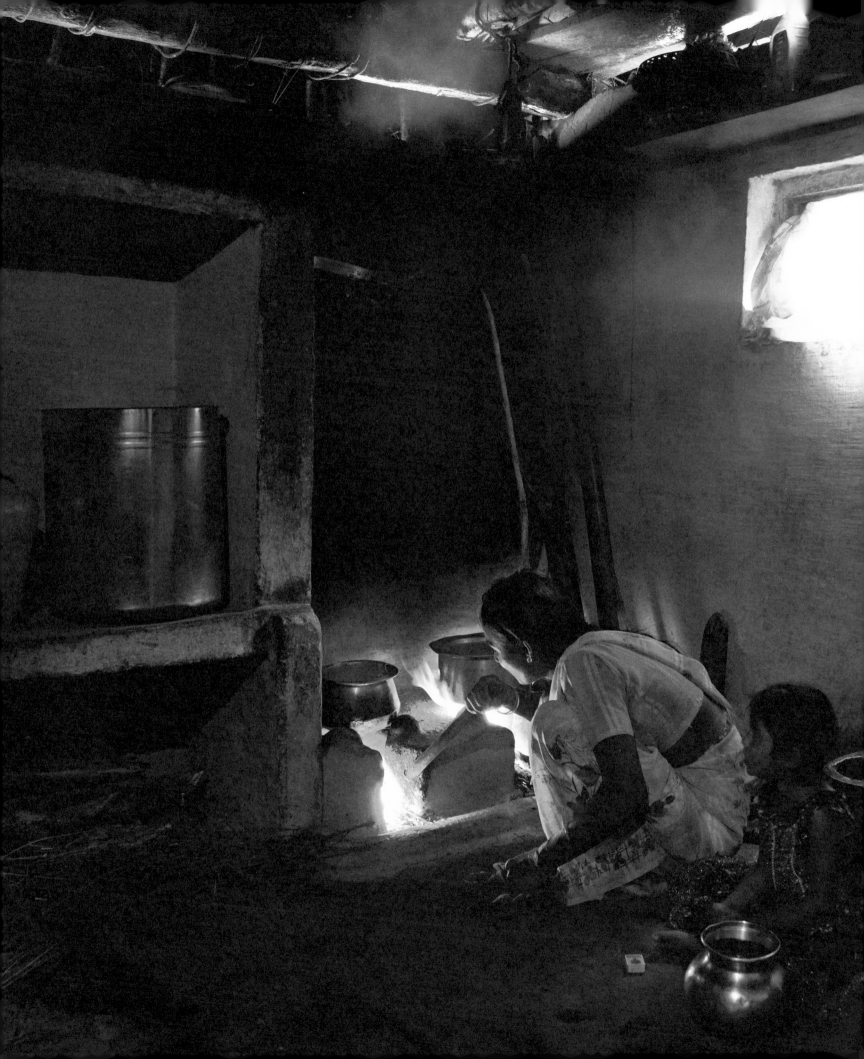

My immediate reaction to this fact—that a man in an off-the-grid village, living without electricity, has invested in alternative technologies to power his cell phone without any government subsidies—was, *How cool! That is innovation.*

Then it occurred to me that he has chosen this particular modernization over acquiring an efficient cookstove or lighting for the home; instead, the household was still using a primitive stove and a kerosene lamp for light, without which the home goes dark at night.

What are the differential social norms that compel this man to purchase solar panels, learn how to rig them to a cell phone, and use them regularly to connect to the rest of the world, but not to purchase an efficient stove that would improve household air quality?

The returns to this household from investments in a mobile phone solar charger were perhaps positive. Noticeably silent, however, was the woman's voice in household investment decisions. Here in rural India (though of course not only here), gender inequality in intra-household decision-making routinely translates into widening and unequal life chances among women, children, and men. Such inequalities and complex human behavior have frustrated governments, researchers, and practitioners motivated to promote millions of improved stoves to reduce black soot, improve the health of millions of rural households in India and elsewhere, and avert a climate catastrophe.

A TALE OF TWO HAMLETS
IN BHILWARA, RAJASTHAN

Two hours northeast of Udaipur district is Bhilwara district. Here, I witnessed a tale of two hamlets that illustrates the complex social dynamics that form the backdrop for dissemination and implementation of improved stoves and cleaner fuels for cooking.

Empowered women with input into household decision-making significantly influence household implementation of sustainable energy systems that ease their burdens on many fronts. These two hamlets—small, remote, inhabited by agro-pastoralist communities—are a striking contrast in their uptake of biogas stoves as a replacement for traditional biomass stoves.

In the summer of 2010, I had visited these villages with my colleagues from medicine and biostatistics to plan a research study of the impact of switching to better stoves on energy consumption by households, and the health impacts on women. During that visit, there was clearly an extreme contrast between the first hamlet, where nearly 80% of the households had switched to cooking with biogas, and the second, where biogas implementation was lagging.

I returned six months later, joined by two students and staff from the Foundation for Ecological Security in Bhilwara. I visited both hamlets to dig more deeply into the reasons for the divergent trends in these two communities.

These two hamlets were separated only by a distance of ten kilometers, were located in the same distressed ecosystems, experienced similar biomass scarcity, and had the same burdens imposed on women to secure biomass for cooking. Women in both communities were forced to walk long distances due to biomass scarcity. Yet by my second visit, 90% of the households in the first village were using biogas cookstoves, compared to only 10% of the households in the second village. Here is a synthesis of what we found after multiple community discussions and focus groups in both communities.

In the first village, which had a high uptake of new biogas stoves, we noticed that an early adopter of biogas from another community married into this village; in the process of moving, she brought the idea of biogas into her new home. Equally important was that other women noticed her experience with biogas, and she rose to some prominence in influencing the others to give greater attention to shifting from traditional wood-burning stoves. This was an important first factor in moving this village to consider biogas as a viable alternative, and provided the necessary evidence that biogas could work in their village. In addition, women became empowered with such evidence (as opposed to hearsay) to make a case within their households for shifting to biogas. As a few households migrated to biogas and provided further evidence for reduced fuelwood collection, reduced smoke, and less drudgery, it motivated many other women to shift to biogas immediately. Continued adoption of biogas in this village was also due to the Foundation for Ecological Security's field team, which successfully increased technical capacity-building in the village to build and maintain LPG units.

While biogas initially was promoted with the help of subsidies, over a period of two or three years those subsidies were considerably scaled back. Yet the last remaining households in this village were switching to biogas, including a young woman in her early 20s. Recently married, she prevailed on her husband to install a biogas unit. She was still collecting wood for use in a traditional stove at the time of my conversation with her, but was waiting to switch as soon as the biogas unit was operational. She was clear in telling me that it did not take much for her husband to decide to switch. He had two compelling forces prevailing on him: his wife would remain one of the few still walking a distance to collect and carry heavy loads of wood, and he would be among a minority of men who had not allowed his wife to switch to biogas.

It takes about two weeks to build a unit, and another two weeks to make the anaerobic digester unit operational until methane is continually produced from a mix of animal dung and water. Under pressure, this methane is piped into the house and is then burned using a stove with gas burners. To be sure, this does not mean that women discard all wood from their homes. While previously they were using 100 bundles of forty kilograms each, they still keep a tenth of the original bundles for emergencies when biogas fails to function properly. It would be nearly impossible to abandon the traditional, tried-and-tested technology of a three-stone stove with a simple wood fire to cook. There is no better backup than a simple stove that can be readily assembled and operated in a time of need. Such traditions are reliable safeguards in households beset with social, economic, climate, and environmental vulnerabilities.

In the second hamlet, gender inequality within households proved to be a key driving factor in the continued use of traditional wood-based stoves in a majority of the households. The Foundation for Ecological Security also introduced the biogas project in this village. Yet its team could not overcome two key hurdles.

First, the team was unable to develop the technical capacity of designated villagers to build and maintain biogas units. Second, it could not get women to collaborate and prevail upon their households to install new units, or to repair biogas units when broken. When women are unable to mobilize resources from their homes to repair minor biogas problems such as a broken valve, or a poorly functioning supply hose, the units rapidly descend into disrepair.

Once methane production declines and the unit dries up, the process of cleaning a unit, repairing it, and reproducing methane is time-consuming and cost-prohibitive. Disempowered women who are unable to motivate their husbands to address minor repairs before they escalate

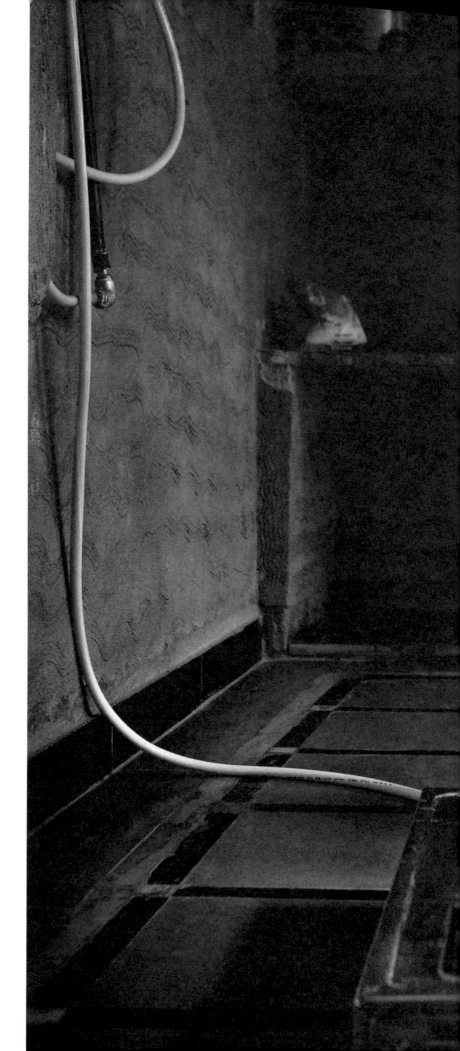

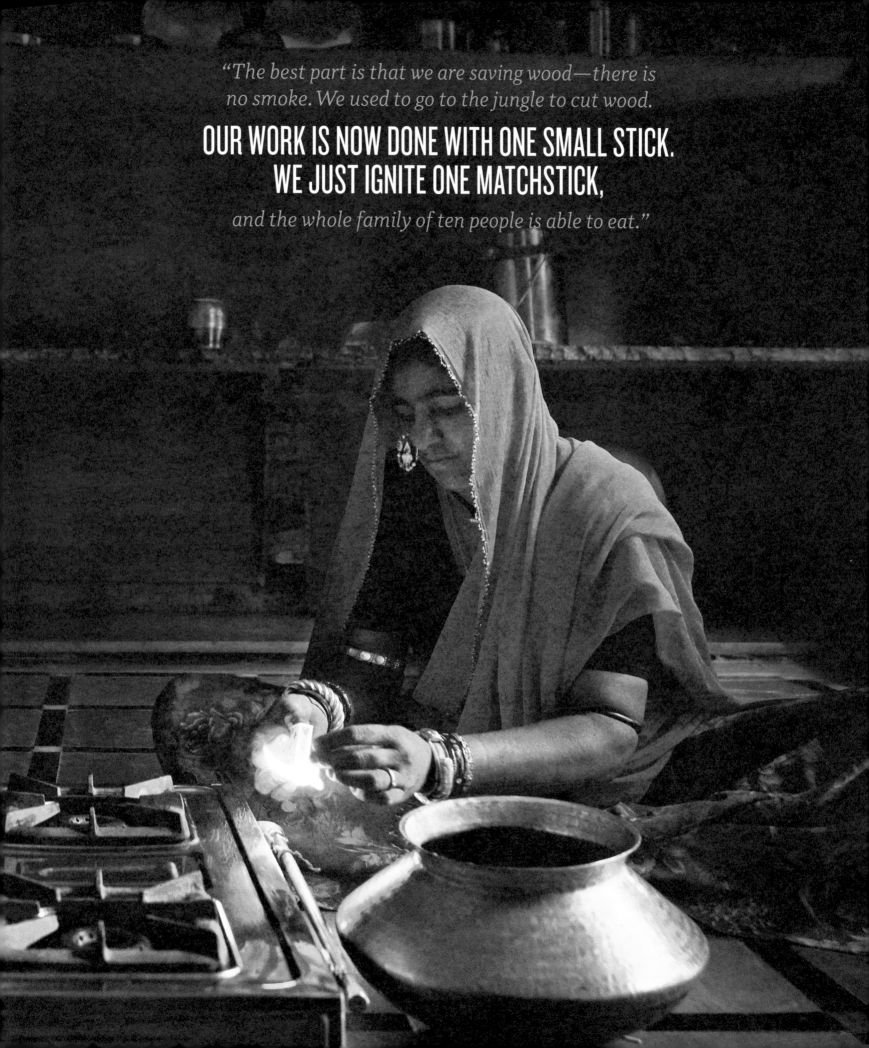

"*The best part is that we are saving wood—there is no smoke. We used to go to the jungle to cut wood.* OUR WORK IS NOW DONE WITH ONE SMALL STICK. WE JUST IGNITE ONE MATCHSTICK, *and the whole family of ten people is able to eat.*"

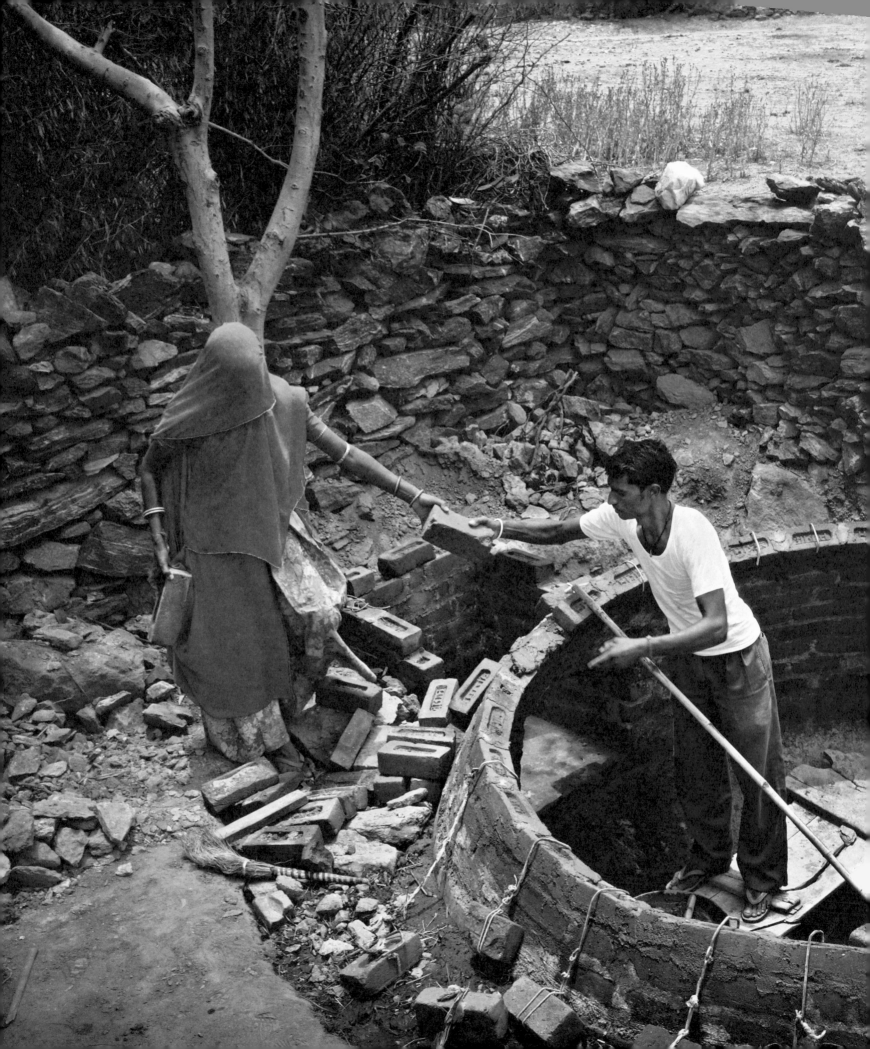

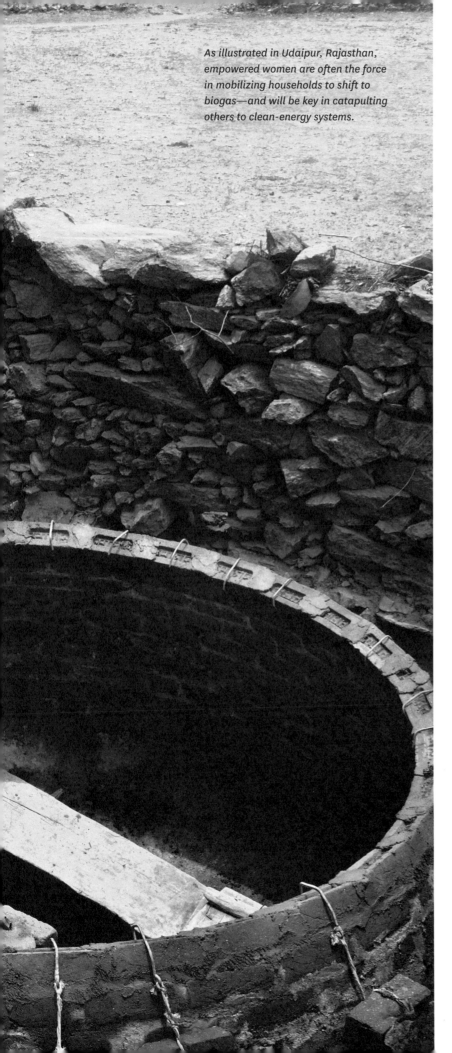

and result in the shutdown of biogas is illustrative of the role gender inequities play in the uptake and maintenance of efficient and clean-energy systems by the rural poor. As units fail, other households have been reluctant to take up biogas. They cite various reasons for the failure, thereby driving down the acceptability of such interventions that hold some promise in reducing solid fuel combustion and in improving household air quality and health outcomes of women and children, who are most affected by wood smoke.

Moreover, in the second village, gender inequities were also the reason for men to remain oblivious to the burdens on women to collect and carry wood for household energy in the absence of biogas. Women's lack of influence that led to failed biogas units also had a dampening effect on the further uptake of biogas stoves in the second village.

Women are central to addressing energy insecurity of the many billions, and hold a pivotal role in the transition of households from inefficient stoves and solid fuels to efficient stoves and cleaner fuels. Only when they are given an opportunity to mobilize and address household energy needs in a sustainable manner are we likely to see the uptake of new energy systems in rural areas.

IN ABDASA TALUKA, WOMEN INNOVATE TO EXPAND ENERGY CHOICES

I have seen many women innovating with new biomass fuels. Given the laborious work of collecting fuelwood, they are open to reducing their burdens if they are able to use an abundant invasive plant species that dries faster and is useful as fuel in the rainy season, or some other plant matter that burns longer and more slowly. Women are entrepreneurial in finding new sources of household fuel if it meets their household needs.

Deep in the Satkosia forest in Orissa, in one of the last hamlets at the edge of the tiger reserve, some women collect the shell of the beautiful black fruit of *Lagerstroemia parviflora*. This, they told me, is hard and works very well as fuel. Women prize this black fuel for its coal-like qualities and slow burning that produces high heat.

This is innovation on the energy front available to women who are operating within narrow decision-making spaces. These small innovations are reminders of the enormous possibilities when women have greater agency in the design and uptake of new and alternative energy systems.

Women have played significant leadership roles in mobilizing their communities to tackle intractable problems. The key is to lower the social, cultural, and political barriers so that women have opportunities to lead in problem solving with their communities, unleashing their ingenuity for the

141

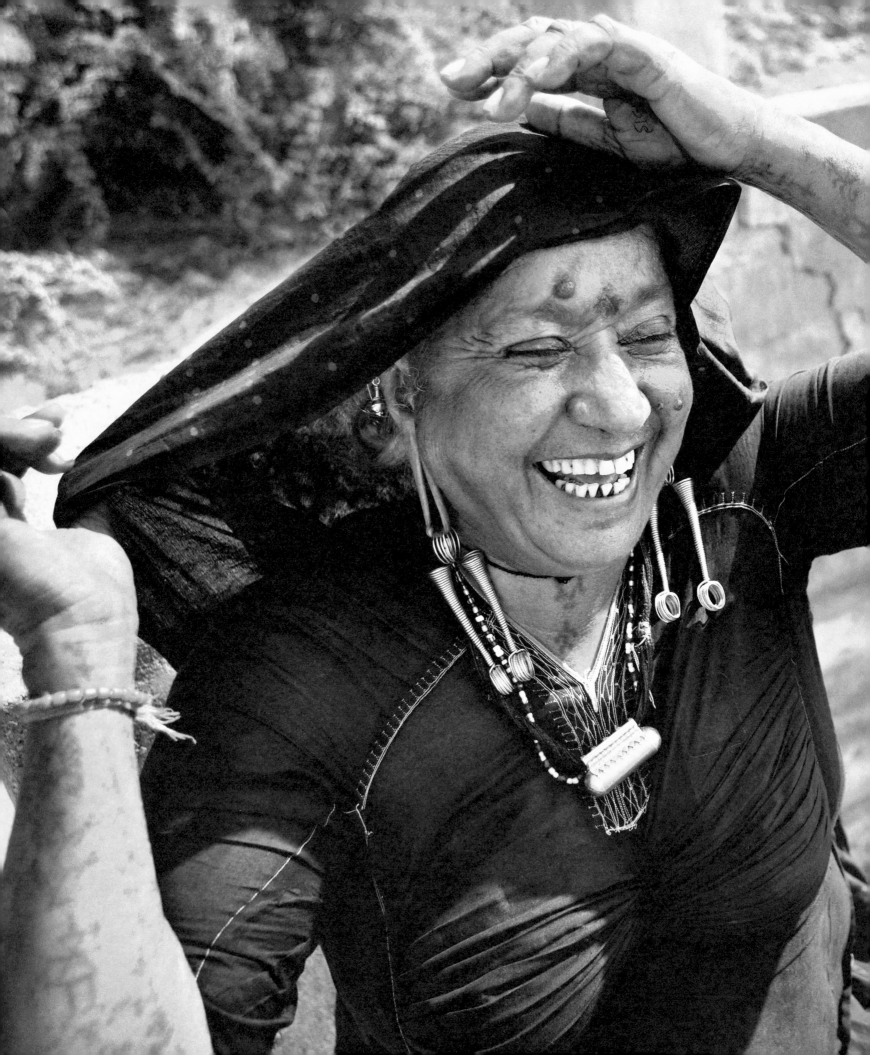

"The greater permeability of women's networks across class and social lines, and women's typically greater distance from local power nexuses, make for better prospects for group action among women than among men."

BINA AGARWAL, *Gender and Green Governance*

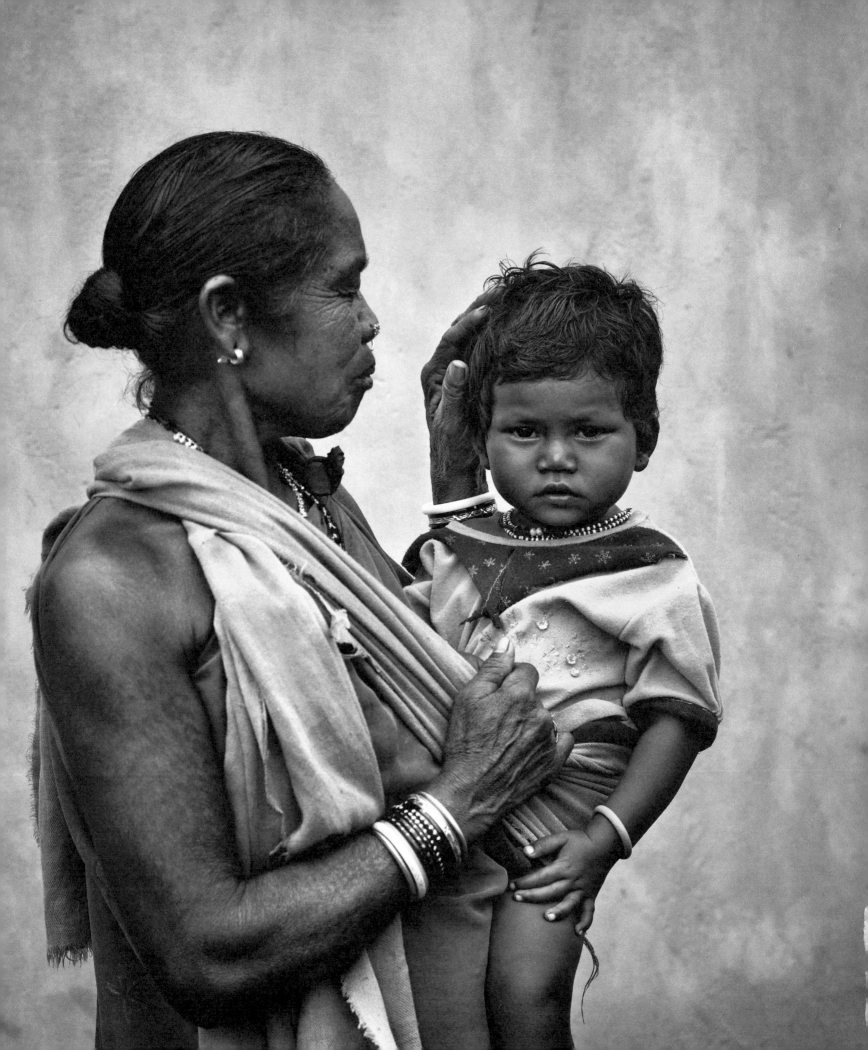

larger good. When elected to a *panchayat* (a village assembly of five elected persons), women have played a pivotal role in transforming their communities using alternative sources of energy.

In the arid desert of Kutch are the Rabari people, seminomadic, but mostly settled now, who raise cattle, buffalo, and camels. In Abdasa Taluka of Kutch, in a Rabari village, I met Hansbai (pictured on the previous spread) through Sahjeevan, a nongovernmental organization mobilizing communities to build sustainable livelihoods.

Hansbai, elected to be *sarpanch* (the head of her local *panchayat*), mobilized solar energy to bring piped water into her village. She organized a water committee, stipulated the costs, and levied the necessary fees per household to raise the funds to install and maintain a solar-powered pump to bring water from a well outside the village into homes in the village. In combining the power of a *sarpanch* with viable solar technology suitable for a remote desert village, she transformed the quality of life for women. Transformative energy systems for cooking will need such a combination of empowered women and communities with agency to design local solutions that leverage new and sustainable technologies.

Sustainability of new energy technologies is predicated on involving people who are end users and on providing those energy technologies that are most likely to last under local conditions. In involving end users, the chances of improving the uptake and maintenance of new energy systems are significantly improved. And vice versa.

In contrast to the Rabari community in Kutch, which successfully mobilized solar energy, an off-the-grid village in Satkosia struggled with solar lighting that was installed under a government project. The Orissa Renewable Energy Department distributed solar lamps at a cost of 200 rupees to households in the village. The department staff also initiated a user association fee of 10 rupees the first year, and

20 rupees the next year to maintain the solar lamps by the community. They provided training at the time of installation but did not develop capabilities through sustained training in the user group to help with the repair and maintenance of solar lamps.

Three years hence, 60% of the lamps in the village were not working. The villagers love these solar lamps but have been unable to repair them, and the government staff who initiated the program has not been back to sustain it. The village was unsure if the solar panels charging the lamps were not functioning properly or if the bulbs were no longer functional. Nevertheless, the villagers were motivated to take these lamps to get them repaired in the nearest market in Angul, but were told to take them to the capital, Bhubaneshwar, another three hours away. That extra distance to Bhubaneshwar would set them back 300 rupees. With no assurance that these solar lamps would be fixable, these villagers from the Satkosia forest abandoned their plan.

A few lamps still work in the village, and are routinely used, but as they break down, there are not sustainable mechanisms in place to fix them. Whether it is government, nongovernment, or market intervention to bring new energy systems, sufficient local capacity-building to support these new energy systems is fundamental to sustaining them in remote rural areas with the most need for such systems.

This is the main reason why LPG is not viable in rural communities. The distribution networks are absent, and the burden is on the user to travel long distances to purchase replacement LPG cylinders or valves for a biogas unit. Even with subsidies, such an effort is costly, and the alternative is cheaper; women and children gather biomass that is in steady supply, readily available, and easily useable. While harmful, it is functional for the household.

And the pattern risks forever repeating. ✤

"I don't try to fool myself that the stories of individuals are themselves arguments. I just believe that better arguments, maybe even better policies, get formulated when we know more about ordinary lives."

KATHERINE BOO,
Behind the Beautiful Forevers: Life, Death, and Hope in a Mumbai Undercity[1]

In 2009, I was in Orissa—the Indian state where this book's central essay began—with academic colleagues and staff from the Foundation for Ecological Security. Our work was testing stove emissions using a brand-new nanoparticle surface area monitor under field conditions. As always, I was thrilled to be undertaking field research that felt serious and necessary.

And yet something pulled at me. In a way, I felt overly bound to this single path of studying stoves. Any larger issues at play—which, as a social scientist, I knew existed—were not part of the project research.

With a bit of worry about where this thought might take me, I began to wonder: How can we think more systematically about this issue of energy use in rural India? What if we pulled back our lens to add perspectives from a range of fields—not just from engineering (Pratim Biswas of Washington University Engineering was with me) but from other perspectives like gender inequality, ecology, and so on? Could there be a way to synthesize our perspectives and present them in a way that showed the true complexity of how these stoves came to be lit, day after day?

Back in the States, at a friend's dinner party in November 2010, I met a photographer named Mark Katzman. We got along straightaway, and Mark took genuine interest in the work I was doing in India and the challenges embedded within it. On the spot, I encouraged him to join me during my next trip to document the lives at the heart of my research.

Six months later, I bumped into Mark again, and it was clear we were both still interested in collaborating. Within two weeks, we had booked the first of what would be two trips through rural India—to interview communities, to photograph their daily lives, to think collaboratively with colleagues...and ultimately to make what was becoming an untraditional kind of book.

> "Science is complicated and often jargon-laden, so scientists may need help from a 'translator' to help tell a story simply and cogently. In doing so, the gist of the message is what matters."
>
> **Alan I. Leshner,** *Capably Communicating Science,* August 17, 2012[2]

WHY THIS KIND OF BOOK—A HYBRID OF ACADEMIC SCIENCE, NARRATIVE REPORTING, AND FINE-ART PHOTOGRAPHY?

We had three central goals: first, to simply tell the stories of the real people behind the statistics and stove programs, people living with dignity on meager resources on the margins of a world consuming indecent amounts of energy. We sought to portray the lives of the energy impoverished—their daily risks and decisions—vividly, yet without reducing the subject to a sequence of heartbreaking images and statistics. We amplified voices and revealed history and circumstances to better convey how household energy behavior is driven by livelihoods, culture, structure, and ecosystems. The practical knowledge these communities have about organizing their lives and making decisions is significant. It is essential that we're listening.

Second, we sought to demonstrate that only after one understands the complexity and messiness of these lives can we formulate policies and design interventions that have a better shot at sustainable success. Perhaps those working within international agencies focused on energy and the rural poor can employ their resources and programs with a long-term vision that recognizes that there might not be a single new imminent intervention or device that will solve our complex dilemma. Rather, I hope to convince some that stepping back for a larger view will indeed take longer, but with greater understanding of the lives at the story's center comes a greater likelihood of long-term success.

And third, we worked to demonstrate that this problem of energy impoverishment—specifically, of cookstoves in rural India and elsewhere—is one that touches many disciplines. As such, solving the problem will require colleagues from disparate departments to come together. I marvel at what my colleagues in engineering know about microscopic particulate matter and the surface area of particles that lodge deep inside the lungs of people when they burn wood to cook. Colleagues in pulmonology are able to test and detect lung functioning decline due to the inhalation of these particles and calculate the Tiffeneau index to diagnose restrictive lung disease. And colleagues in ecology offer a quite different, still valuable, perspective on human and forest interaction from fuelwood use. How can we bring together these knowledge systems and diagnostic methods to engage in applied social science that is directly responsive to large-scale public issues like this one?

> "The purpose of each discipline must be broadened so that being relevant and useful to the larger society becomes as significant as adding to the discipline's storehouse of knowledge."
>
> **Herbert J. Gans,** *Toward a Public Social Science,* February 13, 2011[3]

Those of us privileged to work within a university setting must chart a new transdisciplinary course and make sense of the world anew. Drew Gilpin Faust, the president of Harvard University, once spoke about the goal and purpose of the university this way: "An overly instrumental model of the university misses the genius of its capacity. It devalues the zone of patience and contemplation the university creates in a world all but overwhelmed by stimulation. It diminishes its role as an asker of fundamental questions in a world hurrying to fix its most urgent problems. We need both."[4]

Dr. Faust's call to understand the strength of universities, and by association what we as academicians must do, is most prescient when it comes to examining the plight of the 3 billion energy impoverished—800 million of whom are in India alone. The world is hurrying to act and change, but we have to first understand what it is that we are acting to change.

———————

Following my 2009 trip to Orissa mentioned above, our team traveled to Andhra Pradesh. In a hamlet close to Thamballapalle, FES staff and I asked a group of women about the time it takes to bring fuelwood from the forest to their home and the market. To better understand their thinking, we played a hypothetical game to gauge the extent to which they would travel. As we spoke, we kept increasing the hours it would take daily to collect wood—from three to four, from seven to eight—to see if they would still continue walking such distances.

One woman, when the count reached eight hours, urged us to keep going, saying, "As long as there is smoke in the stove, there will be food in the belly. If we are unable to bear this kind of life, maybe we will go begging in the nearest city."

As we work to expand what this woman considers her options, so must we expand the scope of our own perspectives in understanding the locus of her energy predicament. We have the luxury of making different choices and taking risks. But do we have the will to take collaborative and transdisciplinary risks to make real new options in her life? ✷

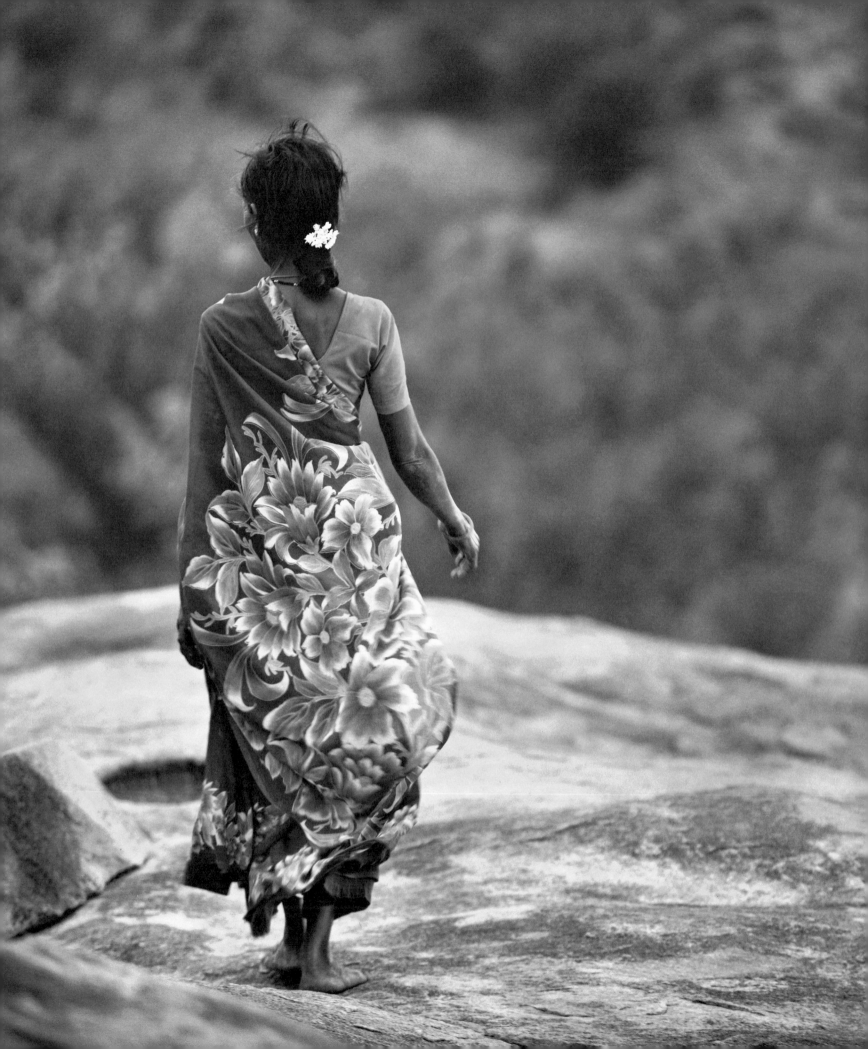

ENDNOTES

CENTRAL ESSAY REFERENCES

1. U.S. EPA, *Reducing Black Carbon Emissions in South Asia*, 2012, United States Environmental Protection Agency: Washington, D.C.

2. International Energy Agency, *World Energy Outlook*, 2011, IEA: Paris, France.

3. World Bank, *Household Cookstoves, Environment, Health, and Climate Change: A New Look at an Old Problem*, 2011, World Bank: Washington, D.C.

4. United Nations Foundation. *Global Alliance for Clean Cookstoves*. 2012; Available from: http://www.cleancookstoves.org/.

5. International Energy Agency, *World Energy Outlook*, 2011, IEA: Paris, France.

6. Venkataraman, C., et al., *The Indian National Initiative for Advanced Biomass Cookstoves: The benefits of clean combustion*. Energy for Sustainable Development, 2010. **14**(2): p. 63-72.

7. Lim, S.S., et al., *A comparative risk assessment of burden of disease and injury attributable to 67 risk factors and risk factor clusters in 21 regions, 1990-2010: a systematic analysis for the Global Burden of Disease Study 2010*. Lancet, 2012. **380**(9859): p. 2224-60.

8. Vos, T., et al., *Years lived with disability (YLDs) for 1160 sequelae of 289 diseases and injuries 1990-2010: a systematic analysis for the Global Burden of Disease Study 2010*. Lancet, 2012. **380**(9859): p. 2163-96.

9. Wang, H., et al., *Age-specific and sex-specific mortality in 187 countries, 1970-2010: a systematic analysis for the Global Burden of Disease Study 2010*. Lancet, 2012. **380**(9859): p. 2071-94.

10. Office of the Registrar General and Census Commissioner India. *Census of India 2011*. 2012 [cited 2012 September 15]; Available from: http://www.censusindia.gov.in/2011census/hlo/hlo_highlights.html.

11. Gustafsson, Ö., et al., *Brown Clouds over South Asia: Biomass or Fossil Fuel Combustion?* Science, 2009. **323**(5913): p. 495-498.

12. Smith, K.R., *National burden of disease in India from indoor air pollution*. Proceedings of the National Academy of Sciences, 2000. **97**(24): p. 13286-13293.

13. Bruce, N., R. Perez-Padilla, and R. Albalak, *Indoor air pollution in developing countries: a major environmental and public health challenge*. Bulletin of World Health Organization, 2000. **78**(9): p. 1078-92.

14. Perez-Padilla, R., et al., *Cooking with biomass stoves and tuberculosis: a case control study*. The International Journal of Tuberculosis and Lung Disease, 2001. **5**(5): p. 441-7.

15. Mishra, V., *Indoor air pollution from biomass combustion and acute respiratory illness in preschool age children in Zimbabwe*. Intern. Journal of Epidemiology, 2003. **32**(5): p. 847-853.

16. Chapman, R.S., et al., *Improvement in household stoves and risk of chronic obstructive pulmonary disease in Xuanwei, China: retrospective cohort study*. BMJ, 2005. **331**(7524): p. 1050.

17. Regalado, J., et al., *The effect of biomass burning on respiratory symptoms and lung function in rural Mexican women*. American Journal of Respiratory and Critical Care Medicine, 2006. **174**(8): p. 901-5.

18. Lim, S.S., et al., *A comparative risk assessment of burden of disease and injury attributable to 67 risk factors and risk factor clusters in 21 regions, 1990-2010: a systematic analysis for the Global Burden of Disease Study 2010*. Lancet, 2012. **380**(9859): p. 2224-60.

19. Misra, P., et al., *Indoor Air Pollution-related Acute Lower Respiratory Infections and Low Birthweight: A Systematic Review*. Journal of Tropical Pediatrics, 2012.

20. Mishra, V., et al., *Maternal exposure to biomass smoke and reduced birth weight in Zimbabwe*. Annals of Epidemiology, 2004. **14**(10): p. 740-7.

21. Boy, E., N. Bruce, and H. Delgado, *Birth weight and exposure to kitchen wood smoke during pregnancy in rural Guatemala*. Environ Health Perspectives, 2002. **110**(1): p. 109-14.

22. Sreeramareddy, C.T., R.R. Shidhaye, and N. Sathiakumar, *Association between biomass fuel use and maternal report of child size at birth - an analysis of 2005-06 India Demographic Health Survey data*. BMC Public Health, 2011. **11**.

23. Baumgartner, J., K.R. Smith, and A. Chockalingam, *Reducing CVD Through Improvements in Household Energy: Implications for Policy-relevant Research*. Global Heart, 7(3), pp. 243-247. Global Heart, 2012. **7**(3): p. 243-247.

24. Siddiqui, A.R., et al., *Eye and respiratory symptoms among women exposed to wood smoke emitted from indoor cooking: a study from southern Pakistan*. Energy for Sustainable Development, 2005. **9**(3): p. 58-66.

25. Pokhrel, A.K., et al., *Case-control study of indoor cooking smoke exposure and cataract in Nepal and India*. International Journal of Epidemiology, 2005. **34**(3): p. 702-8.

26. Legros G., et al., *The Energy Access Situation in Developing Countries: A Review Focusing on the Least Developed Countries and Sub-Saharan Africa*, 2009, United Nations Development Program: New York.

27. Venkataraman, C., et al., *The Indian National Initiative for Advanced Biomass Cookstoves: The benefits of clean combustion*. Energy for Sustainable Development, 2010. **14**(2): p. 63-72.

28. The Energy Research Institute, *Bio-energy in India*, 2010, Institute of Environment and Development: New Delhi.

29. Nagendra, H., D. Rocchini, and R. Ghate, *Beyond parks as monoliths: Spatially differentiating park-people relationships in the Tadoba Andhari Tiger Reserve in India*. Biological Conservation, 2010. **143**(12): p. 2900-2908.

30. Craik, K.J.W., *The Nature of Explanation 1943*, London: The Cambridge University Press.

31. Johnson-Laird, P.N., *Mental Models and Human Reasoning, in Language, Brain, and Cognitive Development*, E. Dupoux, Editor 2001, The MIT Press: Cambridge, Massachusetts. p. 85-102.

32. Craik, K.J.W., *The Nature of Explanation 1943*, London: The Cambridge University Press.

33. Johnson-Laird, P.N., *Mental models and human reasoning*. Proceedings of the National Academy of Sciences, 2010. **107**(43): p. 18249.

34. United Nations Foundation. *Global Alliance for Clean Cookstoves*. 2012; Available from: http://www.cleancookstoves.org/.

35. Smith, K.R., et al., *Effect of reduction in household air pollution on childhood pneumonia in Guatemala (RESPIRE): a randomised controlled trial*. Lancet, 2011. **378**(9804): p. 1717-26.

36. Institute for Health Metrics and Evaluation. *GBD Compare*. 2013 May 8,2013; Available from: http://www.healthmetricsandevaluation.org/tools/data-visualizations.

37. Biswas, P., *Concentrations of particulate matter smaller than 2.5 μm measured from various cookstoves close to the breathing zone*, 2012, Aerosol and Air Quality Research Laboratory, Washington University.

38. Sahu, M., et al., *Evaluation of mass and surface area concentration of particle emissions and development of emissions indices for cookstoves in rural India*. Environmental Science & Technology, 2011. **45**(6): p. 2428-34.

39. IPCC Secretariat. *Intergovernmental Panel on Climate Change*. 2012 [cited 2012]; Available from: http://www.ipcc.ch/.

40. Barnes, D.G., et al., *What makes people cook with improved biomass stoves? A comparative international review of stove programs*. World Bank technical paper. Energy series, ed. D.F. Barnes, 1994, Washington, D.C., World Bank.

41. Kishore, V.V.N. and P.V. Ramana, *Improved cook stoves in India: How improved are they? A critique of the perceived benefits from the National Program on Improved Chulhas (NPIC)*. Energy, 2002. **27**(1).

42. Barnes, D.G., et al., *What makes people cook with improved biomass stoves? A comparative international review of stove programs*. World Bank technical paper. Energy series, ed. D.F. Barnes, 1994, Washington, D.C., World Bank.

43. Masera, O.R., B.D. Saatkamp, and D.M. Kammen, *From Linear Fuel Switching to Multiple Cooking Strategies: A Critique and Alternative to the Energy Ladder Model*. World Development, 2000. **28**(12): p. 2083-2103.

44. Hiemstra-van der Horst, G. and A.J. Hovorka, *Reassessing the "energy ladder": Household energy use in Maun, Botswana*. Energy Policy, 2008. **36**(9): p. 3333-3344.

45. Hiemstra-van der Horst, G. and A.J. Hovorka, *Reassessing the "energy ladder": Household energy use in Maun, Botswana*. Energy Policy, 2008. **36**(9): p. 3333-3344.

46. Masera, O.R., B.D. Saatkamp, and D.M. Kammen, *From Linear Fuel Switching to Multiple Cooking Strategies: A Critique and Alternative to the Energy Ladder Model*. World Development, 2000. **28**(12): p. 2083-2103.

47. Hiemstra-van der Horst, G. and A.J. Hovorka, *Reassessing the "energy ladder": Household energy use in Maun, Botswana*. Energy Policy, 2008. **36**(9): p. 3333-3344.

48. Reddy, R.V., et al., *Participatory forest management in Andhra Pradesh: Implementation, outcomes, and livelihood impacts, in Forests, People, and Power*, O. Springate-Baginski and P. Blaikie, Editors. 2007, Earthscan: London.

49. Duflo, E., M. Greenstone, and R. Hanna, *Indoor Air Pollution, Health and Economic Well-being*, 2008.

50. Yadama, G.N., et al., *Social, economic, and resource predictors of variability in household air pollution from cookstove emissions*. PLoS One, 2012. **7**(10): p. e46381.

51. Barnes, D.G., et al., *What makes people cook with improved biomass stoves? A comparative international review of stove programs*. World Bank technical paper. Energy series, ed. D.F. Barnes, 1994, Washington, D.C., World Bank.

52. Amacher, G.S., Hyde, W.F., Joshee, B.H., *The adoption of consumption technologies under uncertainty: the case of improved stoves in Nepal*. Journal of Economic Development, 1992. **17**(2).

53. Cooke, P., G. Kohlin, and W.F. Hyde, *Fuelwood, forests and community management - evidence from household studies*. Environment and Development Economics, 2008. **13**(01): p. 103-135.

54. Leach, G., *Residential Energy in the Third World*. Annual Review of Energy, 1988. **13**(1): p. 47-65.

55. Leach, G., *The energy transition*. Energy Policy, 1992. **20**(2): p. 116-123.

56. Foley, G., *Photovoltaic applications in rural areas of the developing world, in Energy Series 1995*, World Bank: Washington, D.C.

57. Apple, J., et al., *Characterization of particulate matter size distributions and indoor concentrations from kerosene and diesel lamps*. Indoor Air, 2010. **20**(5): p. 399-411.

ENDNOTES

58. Jacobson, A., et al., *Black Carbon and Kerosene Lighting: An Opportunity for Rapid Action on Climate Change and Clean Energy for Development, in Global Economy and Development at Brookings* April 2013, The Brookings Institution: Washington, D.C.

59. Epstein, M.B., et al., *Household fuels, low birth weight, and neonatal death in India: The separate impacts of biomass, kerosene, and coal.* International Journal of Hygiene and Environmental Health, 2013.

60. Lakshmi, P.V., et al., *Household air pollution and stillbirths in India: analysis of the DLHS-II National Survey.* Environmental Research, 2013. 121: p. 17-22.

61. Lam, N.L., et al., *Kerosene: A Review of Household Uses and Their Hazards in Low- and Middle-income Countries.* Journal of Toxicology and Environmental Health-Part B-Critical Reviews, 2012. **15**(6): p. 396-432.

62. Lam, N.L., et al., *Household light makes global heat: high black carbon emissions from kerosene wick lamps.* Environmental Science & Technology, 2012. **46**(24): p. 13531-8.

63. Hiemstra-van der Horst, G. and A.J. Hovorka, *Reassessing the "energy ladder": Household energy use in Maun, Botswana.* Energy Policy, 2008. **36**(9): p. 3333-3344.

64. Hiemstra-van der Horst, G. and A.J. Hovorka, *Reassessing the "energy ladder": Household energy use in Maun, Botswana.* Energy Policy, 2008. **36**(9): p. 3333-3344.

65. Trac, C .J., *Climbing without the energy ladder: Limitations of rural energy development for forest conservation.* Rural Society, 2011. **20**(3): p. 308-320.

66. Hiemstra-van der Horst, G. and A.J. Hovorka, *Reassessing the "energy ladder": Household energy use in Maun, Botswana.* Energy Policy, 2008. **36**(9): p. 3333-3344.

67. Global Subsidies Initiative, *Fossil-Fuel Subsidy Reform in India: Cash transfers for PDS kerosene and domestic LPG,* August 2012, International Institute for Sustainable Development: Geneva, Switzerland.

68. Green, L., A.F. Fry, and J. Myerson, *Discounting of Delayed Rewards: A Life-Span Comparison.* Psychological Science (Wiley-Blackwell), 1994. **5**(1): p. 33-36.

69. Chapman, G.B. and E.J. Coups, *Time Preferences and Preventive Health Behavior.* Medical Decision Making, 1999. **19**(3): p. 307-314.

70. Chesson, H. and W.K. Viscusi, *The Heterogeneity of Time-risk Tradeoffs.* Journal of Behavioral Decision Making, 2000. **13**(2): p. 251-258.

71. Komlos, J., P.K. Smith, and B. Bogin, *Obesity and the rate of time preference: Is there a connection?* Journal of Biosocial Science, 2004. **36**(2): p. 209-219.

72. Picone, G., F. Sloan, and D. Taylor, *Effects of Risk and Time Preference and Expected Longevity on Demand for Medical Tests.* Journal of Risk and Uncertainty, 2004. **28**(1): p. 39-53.

73. Brownson, R.C., G.A. Colditz, and E.K. Proctor, eds. *Dissemination and Implementation Research in Health: translating science to practice.* 2012, Oxford University Press: New York. 536.

74. Rabin, B.A. and R.C. Brownson, *Dissemination and Implementation Research in Health: translating science to practice,* R.C. Brownson, G.A. Colditz, and E.K. Proctor, Editors. 2012, Oxford University Press: New York. p. 23-51.

75. Rabin, B.A. and R.C. Brownson, *Dissemination and Implementation Research in Health: translating science to practice,* R.C. Brownson, G.A. Colditz, and E.K. Proctor, Editors. 2012, Oxford University Press: New York. p. 23-51.

76. Rabin, B.A. and R.C. Brownson, *Dissemination and Implementation Research in Health: translating science to practice,* R.C. Brownson, G.A. Colditz, and E.K. Proctor, Editors. 2012, Oxford University Press: New York. p. 23-51.

77. Colditz, G.A., *Dissemination and Implementation Research in Health: translating science to practice,* R.C. Brownson, G.A. Colditz, and E.K. Proctor, Editors. 2012, Oxford University Press: New York. p. 3-22.

78. Link, C.F., W.G. Axinn, and D.J. Ghimire, *Household energy consumption: community context and the fuelwood transition.* Social Science Research, 2012. **41**(3): p. 598-611.

79. Axelrod, R.M., *The complexity of cooperation: agent-based models of competition and collaboration.* Princeton studies in complexity 1997, Princeton, N.J.: Princeton University Press. xiv, p. 232.

80. Haggith, M., et al., *Infectious ideas: modeling the diffusion of ideas across social networks.* Small-scale Forest Economics, Management and Policy, 2003. **2**(2 (special issue)): p. 225-239.

81. Dean, L.G., et al., *Identification of the Social and Cognitive Processes Underlying Human Cumulative Culture.* Science, 2012. **335**(6072): p. 1114-1118.

82. Macht, C., W. Axinn, G, and D.J. Ghimire, *Household Energy Consumption: Community Context and the Fuelwood Transition,* 2007.

83. Legros G., et al., *The Energy Access Situation in Developing Countries: A Review Focusing on the Least Developed Countries and Sub-Saharan Africa,* 2009, United Nations Development Program: New York.

84. Pohl, C., et al., *Researchers' roles in knowledge co-production: experience from sustainability research in Kenya, Switzerland, Bolivia and Nepal.* Science and Public Policy, 2010. **37**(4): p. 267-281.

85. Stokols, D., *Toward a science of transdisciplinary action research.* American Journal of Community Psychology, 2006. **38**(1-2): p. 63-77.

86. Dearing, J.W. and K.F. Kee, *Historical Roots of Dissemination and Implementation Science, in Dissemination and Implementation Research in Health: Translating Science to Practice,* R.C. Brownson, G.A. Colditz, and E.K. Proctor, Editors. 2012, Oxford University Press: New York. p. 55-71.

87. Luke, D.A., *Viewing Dissemination and Implementation Research through a Network Lens, in Dissemination and Implementation Research in Health: Translating Science to Practice,* R.C. Brownson, G.A. Colditz, and E.K. Proctor, Editors. 2012, Oxford University Press: New York.

88. Holmes, B.J., et al., *Systems Thinking in Dissemination and Implementation Research, in Dissemination and Implementation Research in Health: Translating Science to Practice,* R.C. Brownson, G.A. Colditz, and E.K. Proctor, Editors. 2012, Oxford University Press: New York. p. 175-191.

89. Nussbaum, M.C., *Upheavals of Thought: The Intelligence of Emotions,* 2001: Cambridge University Press.

90. Cornwall, A., *Introduction: New Democratic Spaces? The Politics and Dynamics of Institutionalised Participation.* IDS Bulletin, 2004. **35**(2): p. 1-10.

91. Gaventa, J., *Towards Participatory Local Governance: Assessing the Transformative Possibilities, in Participation- From Tyranny to Transformation? Exploring New Approaches to Participation and Development,* S.H.a.G. Mohan, Editor 2004, Zed Books: London. p. 25-41.

92. Gorman, M.E., *Collaborating on Convergent Technologies: Education and Practice.* Annals of New York Academy of Sciences, 2004(1013): p. 1-13.

93. Gorman, M.E., J.F. Groves, and J. Shrager, *Societal Dimensions of Nanotechnology as a Trading Zone: Results from a Pilot Research, in Discovering the Nanoscale,* D. Baird, A. Nordmann, and J. Schummer, Editors. 2004, IOS Press: Amsterdam. p. 63-73.

94. Stokols, D., et al., *Cross Disciplinary Team Science Initiatives: Research, training, and translation, in Oxford Handbook on Interdisciplinarity,* R. Frodeman, J.T. Klein, and C. Mitcham, Editors, 2010, Oxford University Press: New York. p. 471-493.

95. Smith, K.R., *Dialectics of Improved Stoves.* Economic and Political Weekly, 1989 (March 11): p. 517-22.

96. Fisher, E., R.L. Mahajan, and C. Mitcham, *Midstream Modulation of Technology: Governance From Within.* Bulletin of Science, Technology & Society, 2006. **26**(6): p. 485-496.

97. Rittel, H. and M. Webber, *Dilemmas in a general theory of planning.* Policy Sciences, 1973. **4**(2): p. 155-169.

98. Rittel, H. and M. Webber, *Dilemmas in a general theory of planning.* Policy Sciences, 1973. **4**(2): p. 155-169.

99. Rittel, H. and M. Webber, *Dilemmas in a general theory of planning.* Policy Sciences, 1973. **4**(2): p. 155-169.

100. Sen, A.K., *Development as Freedom* 1999: Oxford University Press.

101. Nussbaum, M.C., *Women and Human Development: The Capabilities Approach* 2000, Cambridge, United Kingdom: Cambridge University Press.

102. Nussbaum, M.C., *Women and Human Development: The Capabilities Approach* 2000, Cambridge, United Kingdom: Cambridge University Press.

103. Richardson, G.P., *Reflections on the foundations of system dynamics.* System Dynamics Review, 2011. **27**(3): p. 219-243.

104. Richardson, G.P., *Feedback thought in social science and systems theory* 1991, Waltham: Pegasus Communications.

152

NARRATIVE ONE REFERENCES

1. Greere, J., P.R. Hunter, and P. Jagals, *Domestic water carrying and its implications for health: a review and mixed methods pilot study in Limpopo Province, South Africa.* Environmental Health, 2010. **9**(52).

2. Joosab, M., M. Torode, and P.V. Rao, *Preliminary findings on the effect of load-carrying to the structural integrity of the cervical spine.* Surgical and Radiologic Anatomy, 1994. **16**(4): p. 393-8.

3. Jumah, K.B. and P.K. Nyama, *Relationship between load carrying on the head and cervical spondylosis in Ghanaians.* West African Journal of Medicine, 1994. **13**(3): p. 181-2.

4. Martin, W.J., et al., *A Major Environmental Cause of Death.* Science, 2011. **334**(6053): p. 180-181.

5. Wan, M., C.J.P. Colfer, and B. Powell, *Forests, women and health: opportunities and challenges for conservation.* International Forestry Review, 2011. **13**(3): p. 369-387.

6. Nuckley, D.J., et al., *Compressive tolerance of the maturing cervical spine.* Stapp Car Crash Journal, 2002. 46: p. 431-40.

7. Salam, M.T., et al., *Birth outcomes and prenatal exposure to ozone, carbon monoxide, and particulate matter: results from the Children's Health Study.* Environmental Health Perspectives, 2005. **113**(11): p. 1638-44.

8. Sreeramareddy, C.T., R.R. Shidhaye, and N. Sathiakumar, *Association between biomass fuel use and maternal report of child size at birth - an analysis of 2005-06 India Demographic Health Survey data.* BMC Public Health, 2011. 11.

9. UNICEF, *Levels and trends in child mortality,* 2012, United Nations Children's Fund.

NARRATIVE TWO REFERENCES

1. Donato, D.C., et al., *Mangroves among the most carbon-rich forests in the tropics.* Nature Geoscience, 2011. **4**(5): p. 293-297.

2. Walter, K., *Prosopis, an Alien among the Sacred Trees of South India, in Faculty of Agriculture and Forestry,* 2011, Uniersity of Helsinki: Helsinki. p. 201.

3. Donato, D.C., et al., *Mangroves among the most carbon-rich forests in the tropics.* Nature Geoscience, 2011. **4**(5): p. 293-297.

4. Geevan, C.P., A.M. Dixit, and C. Silori, *Ecological Economic Analysis of Grassland Systems: Resource dynamics and management challenges Kachchh district (Gujarat), in EERC Working Paper Series: CPR-52003,* Gujarat Institute of Desert Ecology: Bhuj, Kachchh.

5. Keane, R.M. and M.J. Crawley, *Exotic plant invasions and the enemy release hypothesis.* Trends in Ecology & Evolution, 2002. **17**(4): p. 164-170.

6. Bhagwat, S.A., et al., *A Battle Lost? Report on Two Centuries of Invasion and Management of Lantana camara in Australia, India and South Africa.* PLoS One, 2012. **7**(3): p. e32407.

7. Keane, R.M. and M.J. Crawley, *Exotic plant invasions and the enemy release hypothesis.* Trends in Ecology &; Evolution, 2002. **17**(4): p. 164-170.

8. Lim, S.S., et al., *A comparative risk assessment of burden of disease and injury attributable to 67 risk factors and risk factor clusters in 21 regions, 1990-2010: a systematic analysis for the Global Burden of Disease Study 2010.* Lancet, 2012. **380**(9859): p. 2224-60.

NARRATIVE THREE REFERENCES

1. WHO, *Fuel for life: Household energy and health,* 2006, World Health Organization: Geneva, Switzerland.

2. Jetter, J., et al., *Pollutant Emissions and Energy Efficiency under Controlled Conditions for Household Biomass Cookstoves and Implications for Metrics Useful in Setting International Test Standards.* Environmental Science & Technology, 2012. **46**(19): p. 10827-10834.

3. Mueller, D., et al., *Particulate matter (PM) 2.5 levels in ETS emissions of a Marlboro Red cigarette in comparison to the 3R4F reference cigarette under open-and closed-door condition.* J Occup Med Toxicol, 2012. **7**(1): p. 14.

4. Smith, K.R., Biofuels, *Air Pollution, and Health: A Global Review,* 1987, New York: Plenum Press.

NARRATIVE FOUR REFERENCES

1. Agrawal, A., A. Chhatre, and R. Hardin, *Changing Governance of the World's Forests.* Science, 2008. **320**(5882): p. 1460-1462.

2. Thomas-Slayter, B.P. and D.E. Rocheleau, *Gender, Environment, and Development in Kenya: A Grassroots Perspective* 1995: L. Rienner.

3. Godoy, R., N. Brokaw, and D. Wilkie, *The Effect of Income on the Extraction of Non-timber Tropical Forest Products: Model, hypotheses, and preliminary findings from the Sumu Indians of Nicaragua.* Human Ecology, 1995. **23**(1): p. 29-52.

4. Hegde, R., et al., *Extraction of Non-Timber Forest Products in the Forests of Biligiri Rangan Hills, India: Contribution to Rural Income.* Economic Botany, 1996. **50**(3): p. 243-251.

5. Inter Academy Council, *Lighting the Way: Toward a Sustainable Energy Future,* 2007, InterAcademy Council: Amsterdam.

6. Planning Commission of India, *Report of the Sub Group III on Fodder and Pasture Management,* Working Group on Forestry and Sustainable Natural Resource Management, Editor 2011, Government of India.

7. Groesser, S.N. and M. Schaffernicht, *Mental Models of Dynamic Systems: taking stock and looking ahead.* System Dynamics Review, 2012. **28**(1): p. 46-68.

8. Chhatre, A., *Personal communication with Ashwini Chhatre on Fuelwood Collection and Livelihood Dynamics in Himachal Pradesh, India,* G.N. Yadama, Editor 2012: Udaipur, India.

9. Pimentel, D. and N. Kounang, *Ecology of Soil Erosion in Ecosystems.* Ecosystems, 1998. **1**(5): p. 416-426.

10. Calder, I.R., *Canopy Processes: Implications for Transpiration, Interception and Splash Induced Erosion, Ultimately for Forest Management and Water Resources.* Plant Ecology, 2001. **153**(1/2): p. 203-214.

11. Calder, I.R., *Canopy Processes: Implications for Transpiration, Interception and Splash Induced Erosion, Ultimately for Forest Management and Water Resources.* Plant Ecology, 2001. **153**(1/2): p. 203-214.

12. Pimentel, D. and N. Kounang, *Ecology of Soil Erosion in Ecosystems.* Ecosystems, 1998. **1**(5): p. 416-426.

13. Smiet, A.C., *Forest Ecology on Java: human impact and vegetation of montane forest.* Journal of Tropical Ecology, 1992. **8**(02): p. 129-152.

14. Ribot, J.C., *Vulnerability Does Not Just Fall from the Sky: Toward Multi-scale Pro-poor Climate Policy, in Social Dimensions of Climate Change: Equity and Vulnerability in a Warming World,* R. Mearns and A. Norton, Editors. 2009, World Bank: Washington, D.C.

15. Sterman, J.D., *Business Dynamics: Systems Thinking and Modeling for a Complex World,* 2000, Boston: Irwin/McGraw-Hill.

EPILOGUE REFERENCES

1. Boo, K., *Behind the Beautiful Forevers,* 2012, New York: Random House.

2. Leshner, A.I., *Capably Communicating Science.* Science, 2012. **337**(6096): p. 777-777.

3. Gans, H.J., *Toward a Public Social Science, in Public Sphere Forum* 2011, Social Science Research Council: New York.

4. Faust, D.G., *The Role of the University in a Changing World,* 2010, Harvard University.

153

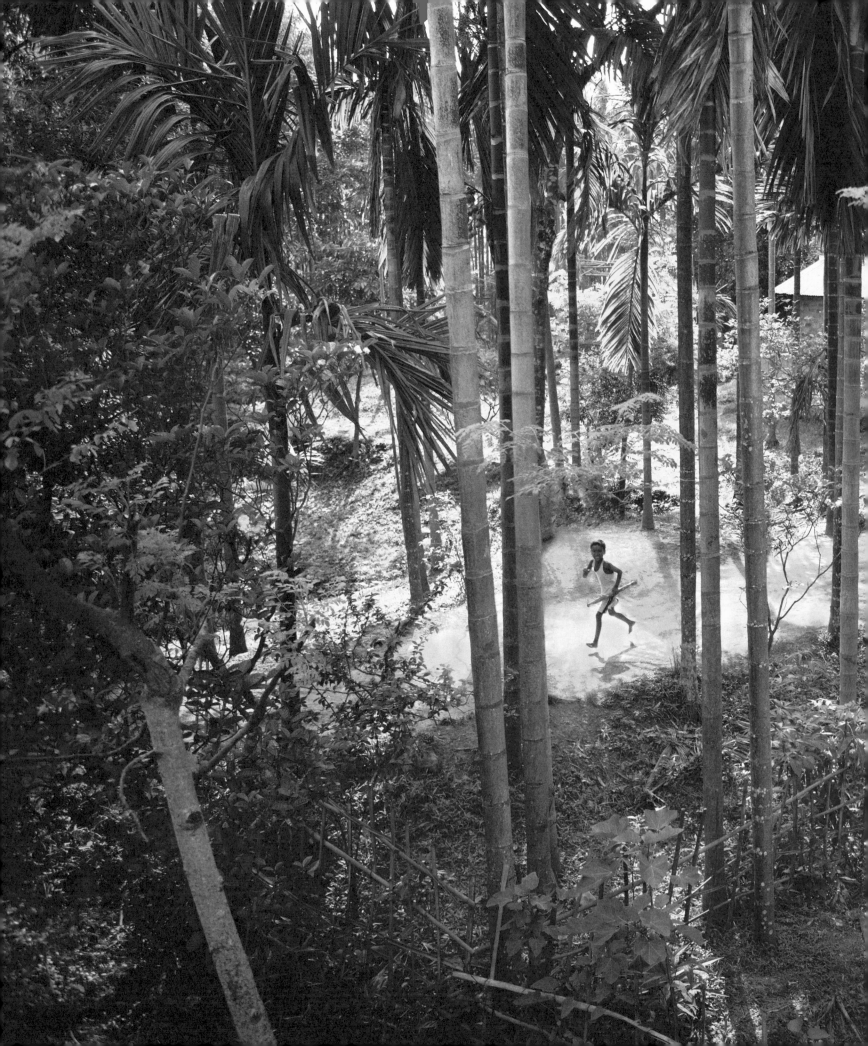

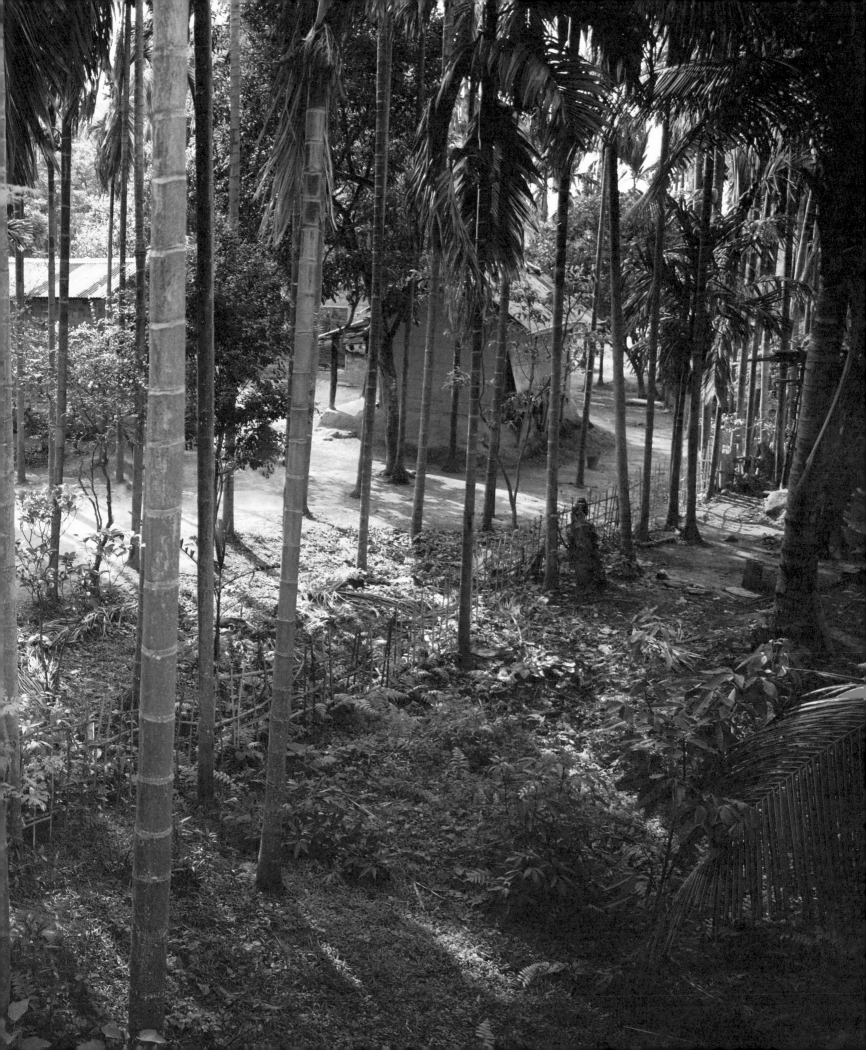

ACKNOWLEDGEMENTS

156

I owe much to many in realizing this book. My Chancellor, Mark S. Wrighton, understood the vision for this book, supported it, and encouraged it, and I am most grateful for that. Director S. Parasuraman of the Tata Institute of Social Sciences; my Dean, Edward F. Lawlor; and colleagues from various disciplines—Pratim Biswas, Tiffany Knight, Brent Williams, Mario Castro, and James Wertsch—made a case for this book very early on. To Amar Bukkasagaram, your generous starting gift gave shape to a book proposal and further support. Significant support from the Charoen Pokphand Group, Indonesia, and Washington University allowed me to go forward with full force, and without that support, this book would remain merely an idea. Thanks to Chad Zimmerman at Oxford University Press for backing this book.

Jagdeesh Rao and colleagues at the Foundation for Ecological Security (FES) have been that constant in all our important work in India. Their input, collaboration, and support of this book are no exception. In particular, I should like to acknowledge the field support of FES teams in Andhra Pradesh, Assam, Gujarat, Orissa, and Rajasthan. Thanks to Bhavana, Gorbhai, and Kiran from Sahjeevan for their guidance and orientation to communities and livelihoods in Kutch, Gujarat. This book had superb research and cataloging support from Colin Whitmarsh, Dessa Somerside Shuckerow, Becca Gluckstein, Laura Olivier, Neha Joshi, Jess Londeree, and Ryan Bell. One should be so lucky to have students of this caliber. With enthusiasm, Nishesh Chalise provided critical research support and feedback. Collaboration with Peter Hovmand on model building with communities over the last several years in India has been significant to my thinking about energy-poverty dynamics. Ashwini—thanks for the engaging discussions about this book. Arun, your work and friendship are a source of much inspiration.

Richenda Van Leeuwen, head of Energy Access at the UN Foundation, was instrumental in facilitating connections with colleagues in the Sustainable Energy for All Initiative and the Global Alliance for Clean Cookstoves. I have been fortunate to get constructive feedback on data and the central essay from Radha Muthiah, head of the Global Alliance for Clean Cookstoves, and from Amy Sticklor of the Alliance. Any errors in data and interpretation are mine alone.

This book is a result of collaboration and friendly debate. At TOKY, I have been fortunate to have Stephen Schenkenberg's editorial guidance, Katy Fischer's design acumen, and Eric Thoelke's aesthetic intuition. At FKstudio, I found an equally driven group intent on bringing the field images of the energy impoverished to life in this book. Paul, thanks for backing up all the photographs, twice, and thrice, and some more after a long field day. Curt, thanks for the magic you have done with these photographs.

To the real magician, Mark Katzman—thanks, my friend, for your sensibilities, pure passion for photography, gigantic generosity, and for your hard work in the field from 5 a.m. to sundown, and then some more in going over the day's work until late, having long conversations about this subject.

A significant part of my professional life belongs to the George Warren Brown School of Social Work. A constellation of highly accomplished colleagues has always set the bar high, especially former dean Professor Shanti K. Khinduka.

At home, the unconditional understanding, patience, and love from Shanta, Aishwarya, Sagar, and Amma make all things possible —GAUTAM N. YADAMA

First and foremost, my thanks to Hilary—my travel companion in life, without whose support I would be stranded; to Paul Nordmann, a solid photographer, friend, and adventure seeker (especially when it came to trying the Indian food); to Jagdeesh Rao and the wonderful staff of the Foundation for Ecological Security for the amazing access you provided our team; to Curt von Diest for bringing the imagery to life; to the folks at TOKY for being patient and forward-thinking; to the leadership of Washington University in St. Louis for your support and belief in this project; and finally (and especially) to Gautam for his ambitious vision, friendship, faith, and contagious, deeply humanistic spirit. —MARK KATZMAN